ALZHEIMER'S MOMENTS

MEMORIES FROM A CAREGIVER'S DIARY

GAVIN DOUGHERTY

ALZHEIMER'S MOMENTS
Memories From A Caregiver's Diary

All rights reserved.

Copyright © 2013 by Gavin Dougherty

Cover and interior design by Sparks & Associates.

Editing by Jennifer Sparks-Bocchino at Sparks & Associates.

This book is protected under the copyright laws of the United States of America. No part of this book may be reproduced, stored in a retrieval system, or transmitted in any form or by any means — electronic, mechanical, photocopying, recording, or otherwise — without prior written permission by the copyright holder except as provided by USA copyright law.

First Printing: February, 2013
First Edition: February, 2013

ISBN-13: 978-1480117471
ISBN-10: 1480117471

For Mother Dear

Thanks to Jennifer Sparks-Bocchino and
Daniel Dougherty for their love and support.

Special acknowledgement goes to all the caregivers helping
dementia patients navigate a heartbreaking journey.

I

EVERYTHING OLD IS NEW AGAIN

Dementia is dehumanizing, like a steam shovel in the mind stripping away life one layer at a time. Each day you forget something new. "Where was I going?" progresses to "How did I get here?" and then becomes "Where am I?" Eventually all of life's compilation of memories, personal history, and experiences are gone. The brain is barely able to command the body to perform the basic functions it needs to sustain it.

For dementia sufferers, their place in the space of reality often recedes over time. As the disease advances, memories and existences get younger in their minds. They regress to childhood.

Short-term memory is the first to go, followed by mid-term and finally long-term memory. In the case of my mother, whom I call Mother Dear, the slide was slow and steady, declining over 15 years. That's the best that anyone can identify when her faculties began to be impaired, her judgment unsound.

My brother Danny had taken a job closer to home in 2001 to keep better tabs on her. At that time, she was able to get along independently although there were a few mishaps like falling down due to low blood pressure, heat exhaustion from too much yard work, or misplacing the keys to her car, and forgetting appointments. It was in April of 2005 that I moved back to upstate New York to live with her and become her full-time primary caregiver for the next four years after a 20-year stint in Orange County, California.

Her official diagnosis was Alzheimer's disease, an increasingly common cause of dementia as our population achieves longer lives. According to WebMD.com:

> *Dementia is the loss of mental functions — such as thinking, memory, and reasoning — that is severe enough to interfere*

with a person's daily functioning. Dementia is not a disease itself, but rather a group of symptoms that are caused by various diseases or conditions. Symptoms can also include changes in personality, mood, and behavior.

The only way to receive a definitive cause for dementia is an analysis of the brain by way of an autopsy. There are no tests for Alzheimer's disease. Doctors come to these diagnoses by eliminating the other possible causes for the symptoms. If it isn't this, or this, or this, it must be that. The uncertainty isn't very comforting but, then again, the autopsy alternative doesn't seem so great either!

* * *

In the middle stages of her disease, my mother constantly asked to get back to her childhood home, the farm where she grew up in the 1930s and 40s. This was the place where she often regressed to when she asked if I was going to take her home. She couldn't understand that home was where we were, a place she had lived for the past 60 years. Home, for her, was her parent's farm and no amount of explanation could convince her otherwise.

She couldn't believe that she owned the house where we lived and all its contents. Her questioning on the subject seemed infinite. She exhibited one of the main symptoms of the disease by repeatedly asking the same question, and testing my patience as a caregiver.

Mother Dear was born on July 15, 1929, near the start of the great Depression, in the small city of Bennington in southwestern Vermont. The area is most famous as the burial site of Pulitzer Prize winning poet Robert Frost at The Old First Church; Ethan Allen and the Green Mountain boys of the Revolutionary War; and the huge 306' Bennington Battle Monument stone obelisk (à la the Washington Monument) with a mid-point observatory where you can see three states. It was built to commemorate victory in a crucial firefight where General Stark overcame British Colonel Baum's attempt to capture American supplies. The victory cut off the lifeline to British General Burgoyne and set the stage for his subsequent surrender.

The area drips with rich history.

Her parents returned home with their baby across the New York border to their farm in the Town of Hoosick. Despite a very difficult life of working alongside her father doing chores while growing up, her childhood home always held fond memories. She was a farmer's daughter through and through and a lifelong member of the Grange. She often quipped, "You can take the girl off the farm but you can't take the farm out of the girl."

As an adult, a pilgrimage to the Rensselaer County Fair in Schaghticoke each year allowed her to relive a part of her youth, strolling through the 4-H displays, barns filled with livestock, and the horse arena. There was always time for the midway, where Italian sausage with peppers and onions, and fried dough covered in confectioner's sugar and cinnamon called out to her taste buds. A bit of fun was to be had by placing a quarter on a color, always green, and hoping to win one of the stuffed animals that hung low over the playing area should the Wiffle ball land in the correctly painted hole after a gentle toss.

When her memory was still intact, taking a drive by her old homestead to see the now-overgrown pastures was something she was always interested in doing. It was there in Groveside where the road turned from pavement to dirt with ruts both parallel and perpendicular, accentuating the fact that one was truly in farm country. We'd pass the place where the one room schoolhouse once stood and her mother taught K-12 to the rural children.

During my childhood, we would drive by her former home and she would point out her bedroom window in the house, where the barns once stood, the rusted barbed wire enclosed cow pastures, and where the chicken coop had bustled with pecking and clucking. There had been a pond where she and her brother swam without fear of the snapping turtles lurking below the surface that were large enough to take down a goose, and the stream where large canisters of fresh milk were placed to keep them cool after tending to the herd of dairy cows was complete.

On today's mass-production farms, animals are given numbers and treated as such. The animals on small family farms all had names. Getting close to the livestock on a farm, thinking of them like pets, can be a bad thing because one day they're there, the next day they're not — being sold or winding up on the supper table. It was particularly common during the depression when money was tight and self-reliance a must. There was Billy the goat, my mother's horned nemesis, which her only sibling Paul would sic on her. The goat would chase her until she climbed up on the rail surrounding the porch to get out of the reach of his horns. She would scream for help while her brother would laugh uncontrollably. Then there was Francesca the lamb that Mom loved with all her heart. Returning from school one day, the lamb was gone. No one ever spoke about what happened, like a code of silence being enforced. It was what it was and she never saw Francesca again. That was life on a farm.

When we became old enough to drive, my brother and I often indulged her with these trips down memory lane.

One stunning summer day, with the temperature in the low 80°F range, no humidity and sunny without a cloud in the sky, she and I embarked on the familiar route shaped like a two-headed lollipop. We would go east about 20 miles up the road from our home in the Town of Brunswick toward Vermont, take a left on Pine Valley Road and drive out through the country to the farm where she had told me of all her adventures as a little girl. She pointed out the hills where she whizzed down the road on her bicycle at top speed towards home.

Then we pressed onward, winding through the rolling hills, leas, and countryside to Hoosick Falls, the home of the cemeteries where our family's gravesites are located. Hoosick Falls had been a boomtown borne of the Industrial Revolution, where a blacksmith named Walter A. Wood began building a reaper and became the largest farm machinery manufacturer in the world by the 1890s. It was later surpassed by the introduction of John Deere's self-propelled farm equipment.

With such manufacturing success, Hoosick Falls became a growing community of opportunity in the 19th century, acting as a magnet for more people and money. It became a regional center of trade and export for local farmers and manufacturers, as well as from the surrounding areas in Vermont and Massachusetts. They would sell their goods and load them on rail cars that ran through the center of town bound for New York City and beyond.

Mom worked for years at the Wood-Flong Paper Mill that was once the world's largest producer of flong mats used by the printing presses of the day. Subsidies to the factories in Germany after World War II led to an environment where the Wood-Flong couldn't compete. When it eventually closed, it was one more blow to the local economy that history left behind.

The cemeteries in Hoosick Falls are where my father and grandparents are buried. My mother would be laid to rest next to my father, and I assume I will end up in the same three-place plot. Kind of creepy yet comforting at the same time. Visiting the graves of deceased relatives has always been a part of our family holidays, a sense of loyalty to our family tree. Growing up, we went to the cemetery to visit my paternal grandfather on every holiday. When I would visit from California I always went there to pay my respects even though I never knew him. Tradition.

First stop on our excursion was my father's resting place. He died in 1992 and was buried on a slope facing the scenic rolling West Hills that are dotted with pastures in the summer and awash in color when the maple trees change in the fall. I was happy to see that the daffodil and hyacinth bulbs that I had planted the previous autumn around the marble head stone, carved with a rose next to our last name, had come up and done well. On this trip, I placed plants up against the stone: an orange geranium, petunia, ivy, and a spike in each of two arrangements that I had planted in plastic pots before we left home.

About 50 yards to the north of my father is the grave of American folk artist Grandma Moses who gained fame with her paintings of the surrounding Hoosick area and Hoosic River. Her works have hung in the White House and been featured in museums and art exhibitions around the world. She lived for a time in Eagle Bridge, a hamlet adjacent to Hoosick Falls.

East of my father's site are my maternal grandparents. Pop died in 1987 after a bout with Alzheimer's eerily similar to my mother's. Grandma was his wife of 60 years and passed away in 1993. We stopped by their grave marker and I placed similar pots of plants with them. Then it was on to the Catholic cemetery down the road a bit where my paternal grandparents were buried. My grandmother had also died in 1987. There we planted the large stone urn with the same plants we'd left on our previous stops.

As we made our way out of the cemetery to Hill Road, Mom asked if we had been to her parent's site. I explained that we had just been there and asked if she remembered me placing the flowerpots by the graves. Nope. Nothing. And I could tell by the look on her face that it made her upset that she couldn't remember. So back we went up the hill in Maple Grove cemetery to show her the plants we had just put in place. That seemed to reassure her and she settled down.

This is another example of dementia sufferers requiring the repetition of events, and every question is asked multiple times, sometimes over the course of hours. Each time the answer went in one ear and out the other, which would lead me to ask myself, "Why do I even bother?"

Next stop was the Alldays & Onions restaurant in Bennington for lunch. A casual dining establishment named for an English automobile maker (1898-1918) sold under the Alldays name. The Alldays & Onions Pneumatic Engineering Co. of Birmingham was a company formed by the merger of the long established Alldays (dating from 1720) and Onions (dating from 1650) engineering companies. Bennington is a Mecca for antique car buffs who congregate yearly for the Bennington Antique and Classic Car Show sponsored by *Hemmings Motor News*.

Making choices had become a problem for Mom. Choosing from a menu was overwhelming and being presented with a multiple choice of the daily specials meant she had forgotten option one by the time she was given option two. Knowing her favorites made it easy for me to select something she'd like from the menu and suggest it for her. My early intervention in the ordering process saved her the frustration and embarrassment of not being able to do it.

For dessert, we dropped by a local stand popular for its delicious ice cream. It's your standard walk-up place where you order at the window on the left, pick up at the window on the right, and then sit at redwood-stained picnic tables arranged around the squat square-shaped building. I bought Mom a hot fudge sundae with lots of whipped cream. She loved ice cream so this was a nice treat for her and we enjoyed basking in the sun, rapidly eating our sweets before they melted.

We made a quick jaunt by the hospital where she was born. She later worked there right out of high school alongside a coterie of girls in the secretarial pool. The young women on staff lived in an on-site dormitory where housemothers kept track of their activities. The young ones would come up with intricate plans to sneak out and go into town during the evening without being caught, leaving doors ajar and stepping lightly on the creaky stairs to make it back in time for bed check.

From there, we started back to New York, passing the Camelot Antiques shoppes and driving by the silos, rolled mounds of hay, and cattle barns of a relative's farm that straddled the border where VT Route 9 abruptly becomes NY Route 7. We meandered at a leisurely pace until it was time to turn left onto a backcountry road leading to Babcock Lake.

My grandparents used to have a lakefront camp and we would spend two weeks there each summer. It was a four-room cottage, painted white with yellow trim, located at the base of a steep incline across from a camp named "Twin Birches." A wood-burning pot belly stove provided the heat on cold nights, with Grandma getting up at 5 a.m. to start the fire so all was warm and toasty by the time everyone else awoke from under their piles of blankets. I remember a large, round, ornate dining room table, a jigsaw puzzle always in progress on a table by the window, and Polynesian-style tiki masks peering down from the corners of the living room. A small sign reading "Chipmunk Crossing" was planted in the yard.

The pristine body of water was always tranquil, no motorized vehicles allowed, and we had fun going out in the rowboat to stroke the oars from one end of the lake to the other. We'd fish from the shore and short wooden dock with pieces of bread as bait on the hook although I don't think anyone ever caught anything.

A sandy beach with a long dock and diving board, only five doors down the road, provided an area to swim. A hotel had been at the end of the lake, long since burned down, cracked cement footings from its foundation left as evidence. It had been a hot spot in the 1920s, hosting the likes of five-time Olympic gold medal swimmer and *Tarzan* star Johnny Weissmuller.

Burgess Meredith, later a star of the *Rocky* films and the Penguin character on the 1960s *Batman* television series, was around during his attendance at the Hoosac School, a quaint and still popular college prep boarding school dating back to 1889. As a teenager, he even dated my Grandma before she married Pop!

We drove the circumference of the lake, winding around bends that hugged its coves, and left via a route that took us in the opposite direction from which we came. It led us down through the edge of the Taconic Hills to home.

Mother Dear was happy for the trip and getting out of the house where she felt trapped. She was completely in the moment for the entire journey. I knew that she'd be complaining, "I don't go anywhere," within an hour and would have forgotten the whole trip. Oh, well. It was nice for the three hours it lasted which was the whole point anyway. It got me out of the house, too.

As her memories disappeared, my brother and I would be the ones narrating these trips with her familiar monologue. I would parrot the stories back to her that she'd told me time and again over the years. The barns were gone before I was even born. I had never seen a horse or cow or sheep or chicken. The pond was dry and filled with weeds. I merely knew where everything was supposed to be and I tried to paint the picture in my mother's mind as she had for me a hundred times. When she gazed upon the landscape, I knew she saw it the way it used to be.

Her life now lives on through the memories of her family.

* * *

It was in the late 1940s that she was old enough to start dating. This was the space in time where most of her thinking was anchored when I moved back home to take care of her. Sadly, we would discuss her first fiancé at length, her pining for him and describing how she would cry herself to sleep from the heartache of their breakup. She had completely forgotten my father whom she was married to for 42 years.

From her notes and our conversations, I know the following:

Before she married my father in 1950, she was very serious about another man. Floyd was a bad boy — a motorcycle driving, hard drinking, ex-Marine that lived in the "city" (Bennington). My mother met him around town while working at the hospital and the country girl was intrigued by his worldliness and experiences in the war. She met him in July of 1946 and was engaged by December. Her parents eventually forbid her from ever seeing him again, asserting that he was trouble with a capital 'T' and he wasn't good enough for their daughter. In those days, children did what they were told and there was respect for authority. They split in February of 1947 and I don't think she ever really got over her broken heart. She held the episode against her parents for the rest of her life.

It was obvious that it was a terrible time for her. Much to my grandparents' foresightedness, Floyd was killed when he crashed on his motorcycle sometime in 1953. It was around this time that Mother Dear suffered a nervous breakdown. I often wonder how that broken relationship affected her early feelings for my father and how he must have felt. In her dementia, and I believe most of her life, she was obsessed with discovering where Floyd was buried and exhibited some resentment toward not being able to attend his funeral at the time. I knew when she was obsessing about him when she asked, "How do you find out where someone is buried?"

Out of curiosity, and with the help of the Internet, I was able to find and visit his burial site in a rural cemetery in Pownal, Vermont. I considered taking her along to provide some sense of closure before she died but decided against it, making the determination that it would cause more commotion than relief.

After she had a brief relationship with a man named Sam, she met my father.

THE MIDDLE AGES

Both avid movie buffs and single, my parents competed for the same seat (last row on the aisle) every Friday night in the theater when the new films premiered. Each wondered whom the other was, arriving earlier and earlier to get the coveted seat. They officially met on the sidewalk outside of Thorpe's drug store. William was showing off his new car and Mom had just enjoyed an egg cream prepared by the soda jerk inside. That was in December of 1948 and they were going steady by May 1949, had a cedar chest to prepare for marriage by June, and a diamond engagement ring by December 1949. They were married on June 17, 1950.

They were an atypical couple from the start but they made it work. Their first test was the setting for the marriage. Dad was a Catholic and Mom was an Episcopalian and both families were active in their faith and church. The Catholics won the day. The ceremony was held in the Catholic church and later my brother and I were both baptized as Catholics although we grew up largely as secularists. As boys, we had no exposure to church except for the occasional wedding and a special day for the Boy Scouts held each year at the local Center Brunswick Methodist church. Our family was very active in the scouting program, both my brother and me as Cub Scouts, Webelos, and Boy Scouts. Mother took her turn as den mother to entertain a troop of youngsters with craft projects and preparations for plays.

Mom was from the "wrong side of the tracks," or in this case, the wrong side of the (Hoosic) river, being a farm girl and Dad was from one of the most prestigious families in the village — owners of the Dougherty Hotel in the center of town on Main Street. Now an empty lot, the structure was razed after a fire gutted the building. The business had been in our family for a long time and my father was born in a room upstairs. The hotel had a bar and its restaurant was famous for open-faced roast beef sandwiches that were popular with patrons in town and those en route to the horse races. Vacationers would find their way to the famous racetrack in Saratoga Springs via Route 22 during August before the interstate system was built that siphoned traffic away from small upstate towns and directly onto I-87 known as "The Northway."

The ownership of the hotel was supposed to be divided evenly between my paternal grandfather and his brother George upon their parents' deaths. George, who had become a lawyer, had other plans and submitted a revised last will and testament to their mother on her deathbed that signed over all the family properties to him alone. My grandfather never recovered from the shock, betrayal, and despair, suffering from severe depression and he was institutionalized in Poughkeepsie, NY where he later died.

After their wedding day, my parents moved to an apartment in Lansingburgh in North Troy near the confluence of the Hudson and Mohawk rivers. Troy was still a bustling city, once the second largest steel producer in the world (Pittsburgh was first). Among its claims to fame are the invention of the shirt collar at Cluett-Peabody, the "Home of Uncle Sam," and Rensselaer Polytechnic Institute. At one time, Troy boasted more millionaires than the much larger Chicago, and their reach still touches the city today with streets, buildings, and parks showing off their names. Large mausoleums of intricate masonry pay tribute to their dead in Oakwood cemetery where "I Want You" Uncle Sam is buried.

Dad worked as a delivery route driver for Bond Bread for the first 23 years of their marriage. Up at 3 a.m. and home by 6 p.m. Within a couple of years, they bought a new cape cod style house in a development built on fields from the Calhoun farm.

After an early miscarriage, Mother Dear gave birth to my brother Daniel William in 1954. It was decided that Mom would be a stay-at-home mother and she gave up her secretarial job at the Watervliet Arsenal. The arsenal was created in 1813 to support the War of 1812 and is the oldest continuously active arsenal in the U.S. It still produces most of the artillery for the army.

I was born Gavin Paul nine years later in 1963, a month before the assassination of John F. Kennedy. I'm told they got my first name from the Irish Bible and my middle name after my uncle, he of the aforementioned billy goat escapades, who had no children of his own at that point.

Without a driver's license, Mom's days were spent tending to

Danny and me, the house, and the yard in which she took great pride.

They joined the local fire department, Dad as a firefighter and she as a member of the Ladies Auxiliary. This membership afforded them many volunteer opportunities, community participation, and a jumping off point to a wide circle of new friends. They attended card parties at each other's houses, set up a bowling league, and performed minstrel shows in the school's auditorium before those became politically incorrect. Mom was a wonderful singer and often had a starring solo, bragging about her turn at *Second Hand Rose*.

Dad was enamored with the fire service ever since he was little. The sound of a siren always prompted him to exclaim, "fifa feedle," his childhood pronunciation of fire whistle. He was elected fire chief of the company for years and treasurer for many more after that. Through wise investing, he parlayed state and town assistance and the proceeds from the annual Christmas tree sales into enough money to buy new fire trucks and construct a state-of-the-art firehouse that he designed.

His responsibilities became much wider when he was appointed to be the Rensselaer County Fire Coordinator. This put him in charge of the radio dispatchers, mutual aid plans among over forty fire companies, and training programs. In this position, he was called upon to be the keynote speaker at many of the fire companies' annual banquets. He was an excellent public speaker and was popular and entertaining. The speeches and awards early in the evening during dinner gave way to music, dancing, and drinking at night. My father never touched alcohol but Mom was known to imbibe on these occasions, sometimes paying with a headache the next day. She loved to dance and spent the nights on the dance floor until the wee hours doing the jitterbug, bunny hop, and alley cat.

* * *

Mom had always paid attention to her appearance. Lipstick and nails. Color, cut, and perm. She would keep up with the latest clothing styles while adhering to her modest sensibilities. Over the years there were dresses of varying hemlines that showed off the length du jour. But what made sense to her were dollars and cents from her meager depression-era upbringing. Why would anyone buy a skirt for $100 when one that was equally as nice, perhaps even better, could be had for $25? Especially when the style had a limited shelf life. A mindset, I might add, that has served our entire family very well — we're a bunch of frugal savers, not spenders.

When she said she walked to school in knee-deep snow with shoes that had cardboard inserts to cover the holes in the souls, she wasn't kidding. I've driven the route she and her brother walked each day and I can't imagine how miserable it must have been. Near frozen extremities in the winter gave way to adventures in the summer where streams teemed with tadpoles, bushes yielded wild berries, and dips and turns in the road made for daredevil bike rides.

In the sixties, I remember her frosted and blond curly wigs sitting atop Styrofoam heads that gazed eerily from their perch on the top shelf of her bedroom closet. Without a wig, she wore her hair long and straight. Her prematurely gray hair was dyed ash blonde in the kitchen sink and was dried using a newfangled salon-like electric hair dryer designed for the home. It was a clever contraption, in a white case about the size and weight of a packed lunch box, which blew hot air through a plastic hose that had an integrated spiral wire to maintain its shape. The end of the hose that wasn't plugged into the base unit was attached to a bonnet that fit snugly over the user's head. Tiny holes were placed all around to let the air escape and keep the makeshift hat from becoming over-inflated.

Her seventies style was about cowl neck sweaters, shoes, and pocket books. Yes, pocket books. That's a term that is a dead giveaway for someone originally from the east coast as opposed to those in the west that usually call them purses. To take this a step further, the colloquial pronunciation is "pock-a-book."

The decade's hair styles went from the Mary Tyler Moore up flip, which switched to the curl under, then to the Dorothy Hamill wedge that became all the rage after her gold medal ice skating performance at the 1976 Winter Olympics in Innsbruck, Austria. Those that didn't have the haircut of America's latest sweetheart opted for the signature feathered locks of Farrah Fawcett from a new television show called *Charlie's Angels*.

* * *

Grandma, ever the teacher, asserted that travel was the best education and we were encouraged to travel as much as possible. Each summer my father set aside his two weeks time off and Mom planned a driving trip somewhere, most often to the ocean, and usually with Grandma and Pop along. The trips weren't always educational in nature per se, but it got us out in the world and exposed us to different places other than our small town.

Our favorite place and location of the most vacations was Old Orchard Beach, Maine. The Atlantic water was shockingly cold but the beach was long, wide, and beautiful, perfect for walking and searching for unique intact shells. We always stayed at the Sandpiper Motel that had a great location right on the sand and near the center of town and the pier. There were ocean trips to Mystic, CT, Hampton Beach, NH, and Falmouth, MA at the base of Cape Cod as well. In high school, I joined the Spanish club on a trip to central and southern Spain.

When I was old enough, I did all the driving on the adventures that were further away. We drove to colonial Williamsburg, VA, Amish country/Hershey, PA, and Niagara Falls, NY/Canada.

My parents went on several bus trips organized by a local travel agency and made their first trip via airplane to California in 1981 to visit my father's brother. Don had lived there with his family since the 1950s. When I moved to Orange County four years later in 1985, I was fortunate to stay with them until I got my feet under me.

Mom and Dad visited again in 1987 when I took them on a surprise weekend excursion to San Francisco. Dad was amazed, exclaiming, "I never thought I'd see the day when I was riding a cable car through the streets of San Francisco!" We did all the touristy things: Fisherman's Wharf, Ghirardelli Square, and Chinatown. At the top of my father's list of things to see was Muir Woods across the Golden Gate Bridge in Marin County where he marveled at the size of the redwood trees.

We stayed at the stately, historic St. Francis Hotel on Union Square. It was on our first day that my father called my hotel room (next door) with breathless excitement. "The Queen is here!" We should have been so lucky. The hotel was broadcasting a rerun of a previous visit of Queen Elizabeth II on the in-hotel promotional channel. Dad thought it was happening real time. What an adventure!

* * *

Mom went back into the workforce in the eighties so there was a lot of shopping for pantsuits, skirts, sweaters, professional attire, and jewelry. The jewelry had to be 'snazzy' and earrings were clip-ons since she never had her ears pierced. It was during this phase of her life that her hair became more important with regular trips to the hairdresser. A professional now did applications of the color and body waves provided volume to her fine hair.

Her first foray back to work was a disaster. She was hired to be the secretary to the superintendent of the local Brittonkill Central School District. He ruled the office like a tyrant, relishing his ability to cause upset among the staff, administration, and faculty, creating a work environment rife with politics, abuse, and harassment.

Escaping from there and leaving her anxiety behind, she ventured on to Hudson Valley Community College where she worked in the secretarial pool transcribing professors' dictation on a Dictaphone. The job introduced her to new mechanisms, and typewriters with magnetic memory cards before the advent of Microsoft Word.

Her next position, and longest held, was at Rensselaer Polytechnic Institute, a world-renowned engineering university. Beginning as the secretary to the operational head of the Physics Department, she went on to lead the entire department's secretarial staff, before accepting the position of secretary to the Physics Chairman.

After all this time, she still didn't have her driver's license, needing to be dropped off and picked up by my father. It was when I turned 16 that she made a personal vow to take lessons and she got her license before me. It worked out well and her first car was a spritely gold-ish green AMC Hornet that served us both well.

Dad worked odd jobs that used the carpentry skills that he had acquired on the GI Bill after serving in World War II. He hadn't waited to be drafted for the war; he'd volunteered and was enlisted in the Army Air Corp (renamed the Air Force) repairing aircraft in Foggia, Italy. We still have the Lire currency and medals he kept as souvenirs.

After his job as fire coordinator, he sold home windows and aluminum siding at Montgomery Wards, and construction materials at Pollock's Home Center where he worked until he retired. His Type 2 diabetes had taken its toll and rendered him partially blind despite the laser treatments to cauterize the bleeding blood vessels of his retinas. His heart disease was advanced, leading to a massive heart attack resulting in his death at age 69.

Mom long resented the fact that he had not altered his diet one bit and left her alone in her golden years.

* * *

I was 30 years old when I made a pact with myself that I was going to come out of the closet on my next visit home.

Mother Dear sensed that something was weighing heavily on my mind and she knew what it was. After many tears on my part, and many assurances that she would still love me no matter what on her part, I blurted out, "I'm gay!"

Mom had already figured it out and acted as if it was no big deal. She was true to her word, life went on like it always had and future talks of dating men were treated the same as if I was talking about women. It was the greatest gift she ever gave me.

She asked if I thought my father knew before he died. I said I wasn't sure if he knew but was sure he had thought about it. I had called the firehouse to ask him a question one meeting night. The man who answered the phone handed it to my dad and told him it was his "faggot son" on the line. Those types of remarks make you think. Dad wasn't exactly thrilled when I came home with my brown hair dyed blonde, either. He was almost blind by the time I came home with a pierced ear!

* * *

Mom's shopping of the nineties shifted from clothing for work to various collections. She retired after my father passed away so negotiating at flea markets and going to craft shows became a hobby. Her house was filled with several collections: paintings and collective plates featuring wolves covered the walls, statuettes of clowns decorated the counters and practically every horizontal surface, cut glass decanters stood on the steps going upstairs, and vinegar cruets had a special shelving unit all to themselves. Stuffed animals, mostly teddy bears, were scattered throughout the house to keep her company, and silk flower arrangements filled what nooks and crannies remained.

She accumulated four closets and two dressers full of clothing representing six decades, and a house filled with her weekend-gathered treasures. I should point out that she was not a hoarder, as this description might suggest, with her home decorated in a tasteful grandmotherly way.

What was so important at the time was eventually forgotten. You can't take it with you, and sometimes you can't even remember it's yours.

EARLY SIGNS

We've racked our brains trying to pinpoint exactly when her memory loss started. There seems to be a notable string of events that are directly attributed to memory loss, others that could be dementia related, or simply forgetfulness from getting older. Who hasn't misplaced their car keys?

Doctors' appointments. Hair appointments. Nail appointments. Chiropractor appointments. Dentist appointments. Massage appointments. Therapist appointments. It became increasingly difficult for Mom to keep track, showing up confused for appointments that didn't exist or were at a different date and time.

Mother Dear visited me in California in 1997. I had my doubts on whether she could make it or not on her own. She made it, complete with a plane change in the multi-concourse United Airlines terminal at Chicago's huge O'Hare airport.

On our way to dinner at an oceanside restaurant in Laguna Beach one evening, a man stepped off the curb into the street, and it appeared that he was going to continue walking directly in front of our car on Pacific Coast Highway. Mom exclaimed, "Watch out for that fag!" I don't think she even knew what she said. At least she didn't acknowledge it. Jennifer, my best friend, was in the back seat and our eyes met in the rear view mirror; our eyebrows raised and smirks on our faces.

Later that week, Mom seemed completely fine when I took her on a road trip to Las Vegas to celebrate Mother's

Day. Our trek across the desert on I-15 was primarily to see Siegfried and Roy's infamous magic show with its white tigers. They had been at the top of her bucket list. I booked our stay at the Mirage Hotel, my favorite place in Vegas, which allowed me to get priority seating at the show. Mom was amazed throughout, sitting in the third row, staring wide-eyed at the amazing animals and trying to figure out how the stunts and tricks were performed.

Mom called my brother and told him that she'd fallen in the bathroom and couldn't get up. He rushed the 10 minutes from his house to hers and did indeed find her crumpled on the floor in the bathroom. Trying to lift her was like lifting dead weight. Dan carried her into bed and sat with her until she felt better.

On his way out the door, he noticed the portable phone was in the breezeway. When he asked her how she had fallen in the bathroom yet used the phone out in the other room, she told him she went back to the bathroom so he'd know where to find her. She'd fallen, gotten up to make the call, then gone back to the bathroom and lied down.

She stopped calling me. I wondered why I was expected to call her each time instead. "Call me collect," she'd say. After a fair amount of time, it dawned on me that she had lost the capability to dial the phone. This loss of knowledge then expanded to the inability to answer the phone. Communication via phone became a process of me leaving a message on the answering machine, and my brother calling back and handing her the phone when he stopped by and discovered my missed call.

The level of the conversation was directly related to how she was doing mentally. If she was confused, most of our talk revolved around her cat. It would feel like she didn't know who I was, just a stranger at the other end of the line.

The knowledge for operating relatively simple devices

escaped her. Buttons and switches became too confusing. In addition to the phone, we had noticed difficulty when the VCR and remote control for the television vexed her.

She could remember that she'd done the same thing every day for years, programming the VCR to tape *The Young and the Restless* while she was at work and then catching up with the shenanigans of Victor Newman and the other residents of Genoa City in the evening. This had become a habit and she continued the practice when she retired. However, there came a time when she wasn't able to operate the VCR at all. That also left the fifty or so movies she'd purchased through a video club unwatchable.

My niece wrote out simple, detailed, step-by-step instructions but she wasn't able to follow them, becoming exasperated to the point of tears. The first step in her dysfunction was the inability to do something she once did every day. The second step was the inability to follow explicit instructions on how to complete that same task.

The frustration of not being able to do things was compounded by the fact that she remembered she could do them at one point. This was a hard stage of the disease because she was capable of understanding that her mind was failing.

Around the same time, she forgot how to use the stove and toaster oven, leaving the electrical coils burning bright orange while she moved on to something else. She would turn them on and forget about them; it's a miracle that she didn't burn down the house. My brother cleverly unplugged the appliances for safety purposes. She was able to use the microwave with a dial-style timer that would shut it off automatically. For a time, that allowed her to heat frozen dinners and she ate a lot of prepared salads from the refrigerator.

My partner and I planned to see her on a visit to New York. The trip was broken up into three parts. We would be with my mother on two consecutive weekends for Christmas and New Year's while we would spend the middle of the week in New York City visiting with friends Adrian and Andrew who would be there from London.

Before we even started the trip, she was confused, getting her wires crossed and thinking that we were both going to move in with her instead of merely visiting. While we were in NYC mid-week, she had forgotten that we'd already been there for the prior weekend.

———

Upon retirement, my father bought my mother her first electronic organ for Christmas. She had played the piano when she was younger and had expressed some interest in getting back into it as a hobby.

She took lessons at the music store where she bought it along with about 10 other students. It was the highlight of her week.

Part of the way the organ industry maintains its sales are to teach the students how to play their current organ while grooming them for a trade up to the next larger and more complicated instrument. Mom had done this several times at the same store, growing more sophisticated on organs that were increasingly complicated.

Mother Dear, looking for a bargain, decided to purchase a beautiful new Lowrey Jubilee at an excellent price from another store four hours away in Syracuse. What she didn't know at the time was that it would make her persona non grata at the local music store's lessons. She even offered to pay to attend. Her primary joy and regular socialization had been taken away from her. These unforeseen circumstances left her heartbroken and there were a lot of tears shed over that decision.

She found a teacher who came to the house for years, teaching her every week. It wasn't quite the social outlet that being in class had provided, but it kept her practicing the organ and stimulating her brain.

The teacher eventually stopped coming when Mom started struggling with her lessons because her dementia was getting worse.

I had been living with Mother Dear for over a year

and the roll top of the organ remained closed, the speakers silent. Until one evening she rolled up the cover, turned it on, organized her sheet music, and began to play. I was astounded. I called my brother immediately so he could listen over the phone, knowing that he'd never believe me if he didn't hear it for himself. This was the same woman who didn't know who I was half the time.

That was the last time the organ made a sound.

The car accident remains a mystery. She had run off the road when a teenage girl, making a left hand turn, pulled in front of her. Mom's car ended up totaled in a ditch, and she was rushed to the hospital via ambulance for observation. She was in shock, and the airbag had deployed leaving her with scrapes and burns on her wrists and covered with a chemical powder.

Was she at fault? The girl took responsibility. Could Mom have averted the collision if she were of sounder mind? Those are questions we can't answer.

Perhaps the most difficult thing that needs to be broached with an elderly parent is taking their car keys away. It requires their acknowledgement that they are no longer in control of themselves or their lives. It's a restriction of freedom that isn't easy for them to accept.

Returning from the dentist, Mom had missed a turn and wound up in the middle of the city. Lost, she later told us, she panicked. She kept driving and driving and luckily found her way home via an alternate route. These were familiar streets in a familiar area, yet she had become completely confused.

It was at this point that my brother was able to convince her that it was time to give up driving. She agreed, and he agreed to take her every place she needed to go: appointments, the grocery store, etc. She was lucky to have the support of a family member that ensured all her transportation needs would be met.

Yet she was still obsessed with her driver's license being renewed "just in case" she needed to drive. This gave me a convenient excuse when she asked for the car keys because she wanted to drive. I'd tell her that her license was expired and she wasn't allowed to drive. This caused her frustration but it was easier for me to handle than refusing to give her the keys. Given her mental state, she wouldn't have been able to start the car let alone drive it.

The changes encroached slowly. As in the example of the phone, first it was how to call, then how to answer. For this reason, it's hard to determine an exact time when things actually started to go downhill.

ROOTS OF CAREGIVING

Broad spectrums of emotions come bundled with being a dedicated caregiver to an ailing parent. A rainbow ranging from the awful chaotic red to the wonderful calming violet, all refracted through the elderly prism of dementia. There are the rich rewards of fulfilling a familial obligation, repaying the care you received from infancy to adulthood, expressing loyalty, potentially rekindling a strained relationship, or exploring a mature new expression of parent/child love.

Perhaps the feelings aren't always positive. There could be resentment towards other siblings and family members that are unable or refuse to help, a feeling of being trapped in a constantly deteriorating no-win situation, overwhelmed by the enormity of the task, or anger that financial conditions require that relatives must shoulder the burden of care by providing it at home for as long as possible.

Big triumphs and subtle accomplishments can be reversed by sudden failures and minor downturns. As time marches on, the roller coaster of the caregiver's daily living can jump the tracks when the condition of the person with dementia deteriorates. The dips can be a small blip or an extended steep swoosh that forces you to clutch for safety and support. You're left afraid and breathless when you finally reach the bottom only to look ahead and see the next upswing of the journey. The path is so intricately woven of twists and turns that the future is never revealed until you find yourself atop a crest, completing a corner after racing around a sudden bend, or the world is turned upside down as you rush through a corkscrew.

The mental swings can be days apart, or within seconds, which can be the most jarring. Even in times of accomplishment, this volatility can yield negative feelings towards the person with dementia that shadow all of the positive rewards. They can simmer just below the surface — burn out, depression, anxiety, guilt, resentment, and frustration — and rise to a full boil with debilitating force.

The danger is that the caregiver can lose interest in tending to their ward. Perhaps failing to take care of themselves, too.

In my particular case, I'm prone to depression and anxiety for which I have been under the care of various doctors and counselors for most of my life. I can't remember a time, even from my earliest memories, when I haven't struggled with a constant underlying sense of fear. Fear of the bad, but also fear of the good. Fear of change, and fear of the unknown. Sometimes it's just uneasiness about a given situation, or it can be as powerful as feelings of dread and impending doom.

My tendency is to be a glass half empty type of person. Knowing that, I've trained my mind to try to see the bright side of any situation. I used this tool to cope with being a caregiver. Instead of something being overwhelming, embarrassing, and sad it could just as easily be viewed as interesting, endearing, and humorous. I was lucky that Mother Dear wasn't abusive or nasty, as I've heard from other caregivers about their relatives and clients.

* * *

Preparing to go off to kindergarten, my parents had bought a few new outfits for me. That was big news in our household as money was tight. It was a concern that I was aware of even at the age of four. I grew up in a time and place where everything was of value and was attainable with disciplined saving. New cars were rare and everyone in the neighborhood made their way over to "ooh" and "aah" over the latest big purchase of Detroit iron.

When it came to my new clothes, my favorite item was a robin's-egg blue pair of pants that I wore on my very first day of school. You can tell I was proud by the photo taken of me standing in the front yard, squinting from the beaming morning sun, and holding my book bag at my side with the Eager Beaver pencil case inside. An I.D. tag hung from my belt as I climbed the steps into the yellow school bus. The driver smiled, greeted me with a welcome aboard, and waved to my mother. I was afraid.

The play area just outside of the classroom was what you would expect at a suburban school surrounded by a lot of land. There was a slide, swings, sandbox, merry-go-round, monkey bars, teeter-totters, and plenty of room to run. Clover and dandelions were intermixed with the grass to form a dense green lawn for leapfrog and somersaults.

It was within the first week of school that I fell during recess while racing around the grounds playing a game of tag. A large grass stain on one of the knees marred the pants that had brought me such pride and joy. I began to cry. The playground aide, a woman with a repaired cleft palate and funny voice, consoled me. I told her that my mother was going to be so disappointed. I was sure I had ruined them despite the aide's reassuring words to the contrary. My mother would never be able to wash out the ugly green splotch in the fabric. I stared at the smudge and desperately wondered what I was going to do to fix it.

Childhood memories like these demonstrate how much of our lives can be foreshadowed. Personality patterns are set early. At the time, I was more worried about my mother's feelings than my own. Other boys were tumbling and running around without a care in the world, let alone worrying about how their mothers were going to get their pants clean. Yet I was already taking care of my mother in a four-year-old's way. It was a similar role I would feel at different points in my life and eventually assume full-time so many years later.

A heightened level of emotional awareness came to me in the sixth grade when I was hospitalized with terrible pain in my abdomen that had gone on for nearly a month. During my week's stay, the doctors initially thought an ulcer was the source of the trouble and ordered up a series of X-rays that included an upper GI series. I drank the chalky mixture and watched it move through my esophagus in a live image. The screen was mounted on the drab gray cinder block wall of the examining room. Eventually the diagnosis was stomach spasms that I now refer to as "stress belly," brought on by stress induced by a demanding school band teacher. I was administered Atarax, a medication primarily used as an antihistamine with a secondary use for general anxiety disorder. Not only was I calmer, but my sinuses were clear, too!

My stomach was relaxed and that allowed me to resume eating regularly. I should have been placed on it as a daily treatment. Instead, it was prescribed for the stomach spasms and once those were alleviated, the prescription was not refilled. As long as I wasn't in a crisis stage, there was no medical help. Years later, I was placed on Paxil, a popular Selective Serotonin Reuptake Inhibitor (SSRI) for relief from the similar symptoms caused by depression, anxiety, and social phobia.

This history illustrates that I've been to emotional rodeos before, and while my experiences may be common with other caregivers, my reactions are definitely my own.

Over the years, I have tried to tame the trials and tribulations of everyday life through the marvels of modern pharmaceuticals, counseling, and yoga. I've settled into these feeling like a well-worn pair of dungarees. I have an inner sense of when negativity is coming on, the course it is likely to take, and its degree of severity. However, I never know how long it will last before the cloud lifts. I know it will, and I have to constantly remind myself that I just need to hang on until it does. When it feels like there's no light at the end of the tunnel, the only voice that can convince me otherwise is my own.

II

ARRIVAL

The end of a relationship in California coincided with a worsening of Mother Dear's condition. She was quickly heading towards round-the-clock care. It was this synchronization of events that lead me to move back to the home where I grew up. I would choose to turn back the clock of my life by 20 years.

After consulting with friends and family, and much soul searching, it was widely agreed that it would be a rewarding experience that I would not regret. I didn't know how long of a commitment it was going to require or how hard it would actually be.

It wasn't easy giving up a life that was 15 minutes from the attractions in Disneyland, 30 minutes from the beach to watch dolphins frolic in the ocean's waves, an hour from downhill skiing in the mountains, or tanning under spraying misters by a pool in Palm Springs. I would be giving up two decades of relationships, my circle of friends, business associates, political contacts, traditional Friday nights at the movies, and Sunday evening season tickets for the Broadway Series at the Orange County Performing Arts Center.

I had a good-bye party with my friends, then boxed up all of my belongings and placed them in storage, found a home for my car, packed my clothes in a few suitcases, and flew east.

In New York, I would try to pick up where I had left off after college by re-establishing closer friendships with those I had maintained contact with since I had moved away. Since all contact with my work clients was already via phone and email, I would be able to continue working and have some income.

When I first arrived back at Mom's house full time, she was in miserable condition. She wasn't able to get out of bed until noon, and then it was with great effort. She would be weak, trembling, and spend the remainder of the day in her flannel nightgown after she arose.

She complained of pain and weakness every morning. Part of "the cure" was to wait it out and try to get her some orange juice to raise her blood sugar for energy. But when she couldn't get up out of bed, she couldn't drink the juice and start taking her morning pills. It was a process that took about an hour to get through.

Me: Do you want me to help you sit up so you can drink your juice?

Mom: Don't cry at my funeral. You don't know how terrible I feel. I just wish I would die. I wish I could just close my eyes, go to sleep, and never wake up.

Me: Well, I can't help you with that.

Mom: [Looking at me seriously.] Maybe you could.

After several weeks of similar exchanges, and several weeks of regularly scheduled healthy meals, she eased out of this pattern as her strength returned and her overall condition improved. Her spirits lifted, she got dressed, and her personality became more interactive. Physically she was much better but her mental challenges persisted.

* * *

For a time, if we had an appointment listed on the calendar, she was really good at remembering that she had to go somewhere. She didn't always know what, where, when, or with whom, but it did get trapped in her mind somewhere. Leaving the house triggered her instinct to take a shower. Early on, this was a good thing. As her disease progressed, this process became much more difficult.

I had showering down to a sport. I acted like a coach getting a benchwarmer into the game and giving them directions to get the job done. With Mom, the hardest part was motivating her to get in the game.

To reduce her confusion, the first thing was to remove any cleansing products that wouldn't be used. That meant an all-in-one shampoo and conditioner, a body wash (she liked St. Ives Apricot scrub) and a bar of soap were the only things on the bathtub's edge.

I laid out new clothes on the bed and turned on the water to a soothing temperature. Then I would get her into the bathroom, and close the door between us, leaving an inch wide opening so I could communicate clearly with her while maintaining her privacy.

I'd instruct her to disrobe, step into the tub, and pull the curtain closed. When I heard the metal rings of the shower curtain squeal along the rod, I stepped back into the room to orchestrate the production from the other side. I talked to her the entire time so she knew exactly what I was doing, what to expect, and what she should be doing. I would reach in and lift the lever that forced the water streaming down from above. The next phase of the playbook was instructing her on what to do, telling her to start with wetting her hair, how to use the shampoo in the green bottle, and so on.

Completed, I'd turn the hot and cold knobs off and hand her a fresh towel from around the curtain. I'd return to the hallway and instruct her to get out, dry off, and then wrap herself in the towel. I'd go back into the bathroom, comb her hair, and help her put on deodorant and brush her teeth.

Even on the best days, it was a very taxing experience for her. She'd wander into the bedroom and flop down on the bed, exhausted. After letting her catch her breath, I'd commence with helping her get dressed.

I had to pay attention to the details. During one particular fainting episode, I got her wrapped in a towel and assisted her across the hall so she could lie down on the bed and get her bearings. That's when I discovered she had used the body scrub for her hair. When she revived, I brought her to the kitchen sink to rinse the goop out of her hair and wash it properly with shampoo.

She always sprayed her hair to keep it in place. I had to relocate the air freshener after catching her using the Renuzit from atop the toilet's tank as an Aquanet replacement. All spray cans looked the same to her. It didn't do anything for her hair, but she smelled like a citrus breeze!

The experience helped me realize what things we take for granted. Like knowing what shampoo is. Mom could still read — she read the headlines in the daily newspaper and a little monthly digest I subscribed to about her daytime television programs. These pages were read over and over again because while she could read, she had no ability to comprehend or retain any of it. This played a part in not being able to understand that the shampoo bottle said "shampoo" on it. And you would think that the grit of the body scrub would alert her that it wasn't shampoo. After all, she'd been washing her hair all her life. But her brain didn't make those connections.

The brain is a wonderfully complex thing and amazing when it's healthy. Enjoy life while you can. Living with Mom and seeing her troubles made it easier for me to really understand the phrase, "Stop and smell the roses."

* * *

Over the years, Mom became more and more averse to taking a shower. The shower was the most stressful thing in her life. The water bothered her, the confined space bothered her, the faucet and shower head bothered her, and the confusion on which cleansing products to use bothered her. Even with explicit step-by-step guidance, there was anxiety around what exactly she was supposed to do when she got into the tub.

There had been times when it had caused so much anxiety that she got so weak she collapsed on the bathroom floor in a heap before she even took off her clothes. I would have to get her up and to the bed. With such an extreme reaction, I understood why she avoided it.

Yes, yes, yes. We did what we could to mitigate her fears. Dan bought a special plastic chair for the shower so she could sit and wash (she hated it), suggested clear shower doors instead of a curtain (she hated change more than showering), and switched to a shower wand so she could have more control of the water (she didn't understand it). We removed them shortly thereafter because they made things worse, confusing her even more, the tools being a hindrance rather than a help.

I began to let a longer time lapse between showers, often waiting for her to develop body odor, before I would put her through the ordeal. Most times it would take a great deal of negotiation and sternness to get her to agree.

I would let loose with a silent "WooHoo" when she occasionally came up with the idea to shower and did it on her own with no harping or nagging. I would set out the towel, explain the soap and shampoo, tell her to start with her head and work down, started the water to get it warm, and away she would go. Those were the easy times when she was able to get dressed with the nice clean under clothes, shirt, and pants I had set out for her.

This may not seem like much of an exciting thing, but trust me, it was. Those were the good days!

Oddly enough, if she was going to shower without my help she preferred to do it when I wasn't home. One night I went grocery shopping and the deed was done when I got home. A week later, when I returned from the market, I thought she had showered. I asked her, and she replied, "Yes." I went into the bathroom to put away a new multi-pack of soap and there were no wet towels and no residual humidity. I called her on it and she laughed. "I didn't think you'd go so far as to check!" While the answer wasn't in the positive, I did give her some credit that her brain was able to anticipate my reaction and lie about it.

* * *

She had several services in place to help with the chores around the house.

- Paula, a neighbor, had been cleaning the house for over 25 years. It was difficult to tell her that her services were no longer needed, as I'd be taking over those duties. She had watched the slow downward spiral that had taken place every week, three hours at a time — first with my father, whose 30-year battle with diabetes resulted in years of blindness before his death — and then with my mother. Paula did more than clean. She was a friend and often checked on Mom to make sure she'd eaten and taken her pills.
- The lawn care company would fertilize and maintain the health of the grass by making sure there were no pests. Grubs decimate lawns in this area by munching on the grass's roots. The most effective control is to chemically treat the sod. Mom spent lavishly on her prized yard and gardens.
- Jim and Rose had mowed the lawn since I moved away in 1985. I kept them on when I returned since my mother's lawnmower found a home somewhere else along the way and they had been very good to my mother: understanding, patient, caring, hard working, and never taking advantage. I decided that if I were going to spend time in the yard, I'd rather spend it planting flowers in the gardens as a joyful stress reliever rather than mowing the grass as an additional chore.

- Lastly, there was Terry the exterminator. Carpenter ants had been in the house since I was a tyke and Mom eventually hired professionals to come in and get rid of them once and for all. The process was successful and we'd kept the company on for maintenance and vector control. I didn't mind catching chipmunks in Have-a-Heart traps and then letting them go in the woods nearby but there's one thing I have no interest in doing, and that's removing dead mice from traps. Our cats were interested in hunting for moles and birds in the yard but refused to catch anything in the basement. Perhaps it was the lack of a challenge.

The story of the exterminator is interesting and illustrates one of the positive things about living in a small, tight-knit community where everyone seemingly knows each other. It turned out that Terry was the son of my mother's childhood best friend. The two girls had grown up on neighboring acreages and had weekly sleepovers, went swimming in the pond at Mom's house, and took a dip in the river near her house.

Despite all the things that Mom had forgotten, she always lit up like a bright star when he arrived for his quarterly pre-arranged appointments. Mom knew him and that he was somehow connected to her pal, but she kept confusing him as her friend's husband rather than her son.

He would tell his mother we were on his schedule and she always sent her best regards. In return, Mom would insist that he tell her to stop by the house and spend an afternoon catching up on old times. Unfortunately, she lived a half hour away and it was too much for her to make the trip.

One thing I discovered is the number of people who stayed away because they didn't "want to see her like that." I'm not sure if this was because they were concerned for her, really concerned about seeing a potentially scary ending for themselves, or both.

ENDEARING ADVENTURES

As the sayings go, "Every cloud has a silver lining," "Look on the bright side," and "Find the humor in everything." These are mantras that caregivers need to chant in their minds.

Once a year, the company that held my mother's Long-Term Healthcare insurance policy sent a letter to her primary care physician asking for an update on her current medical status. The insurance company would also contract with an independent nurse to make a house call to ask a set of general questions about her physical capabilities and mental awareness, assess her needs, and then provide them with a report. The interviews took about an hour.

The standard questioning always put Mom in a foul mood. She would become frustrated and angry when I answered the nurse's questions in a truthful way because she believed that she was more capable than she was in reality. It sounded offensive to her when I told the nurse that she wasn't able to do certain simple things. In her mind, she could do these trivial tasks. Except when it came to doing them, she couldn't. She thought she could drive the car but wouldn't be capable of unlocking the door.

She wasn't able to answer the questions herself. When a doctor asked how she was feeling during an appointment, she'd turn to me to provide the answer. It would become a triangular conversation with a common refrain of, "Ask him. He knows better than I do."

As Mom sat and listened to my responses to the nurse, I said that she needed help fixing her dinner, getting in and out of the shower, etc. Because she thought she could do all of those things, she scowled and complained that I was lying. And, not only was I lying, but I was telling them to a stranger. These things were clearly no one's business but her own. I was lucky that she would forget the conversation as soon as the nurse left so there was no holding it against me.

The interview continued and I was asked about our shower set up. I responded that we had a shower chair, hand held shower wand, and a grip bar to facilitate her bathing.

Mom: [Miffed.] Well, I'd like to see that.

I jumped at the opportunity and brought her into the bathroom and showed her. Of course, it didn't register.

I decided to try a different tactic when we returned to the living room and resumed the questioning. I tried to involve her more in the answers to see if that would cause less irritation.

Nurse: Does she have any signs of arthritis?

Me: [To Mom.] Why don't you hold up your hands and show her your fingers?

Mom liked to show off her fingers with their crooked knuckles from arthritis. Normally she was proud of them. They were a badge of honor from decades of taking dictation as a stenographer and typing as a secretary.

But not on that day. Mom sneered as she raised her middle finger and flipped the bird to the nurse.

In the earlier years, she could still perform the math portion of the quizzes. That was great news at that point. A section of the interview involved basic arithmetic and logic. The nurse asked her to subtract 3 from 17. If she was correct, she was asked to subtract 3 from the result. Mom went to 14, to 11, to 8, to 5, and to 2 when the question ended.

I was really proud of her. Go Mom!

* * *

During Lent, the supermarket carried Polish confections called Paczki (Germans call them Berliners and Austrians call them Krapfen). There is a rather large Polish and Ukrainian community that settled in the area around the turn of the 20th century. Paczkis are essentially jelly doughnuts by another name. They are covered with confectioner's sugar or glaze with fruit jam or crème filling in the center.

Mom had a bit of a sweet tooth and these were tailor made for her. Not only did they look and taste delicious, they were easy to fix — you opened the box and grabbed one! Mother Dear came into the den with a messy powdered sugar moustache after biting into a Paczki. They're rather large and she asked me to cut it in half for her. I did, and she finished it up.

In addition to her face being transformed into a white sugar pie, she had raspberry jelly all over her chin. It was too cute. I began to giggle and that got her giggling. After a good-natured laugh, I took the plate into the kitchen and returned with a damp paper towel to clean her up.

* * *

Mother Dear always complained that she was freezing. Sometimes I wondered if it was all in her imagination, but if she touched you with her hand, you just about leaped out of your skin because it was so startlingly cold. I've learned that as we get older, our skin gets thinner, and that's the reason so many of the elderly complain of the temperature — both hot and cold.

Mom: It's freezing in here. I wish I knew where I could get some heat.

I went over to check the thermometer. It seemed pretty comfortable in the house to me; I had bumped up the setting on the thermostat when the temperature outside had dropped below 10°F.

Me: It says it's 70 degrees in here.

Mom: Bullshit!

Me: Oh, so you're right and the thermometer is wrong.

Mom: Don't get smart with me.

Me: You started it.

Yes, sometimes I allowed myself to get pulled down to the level of a schoolyard argument. So there.

* * *

There was a lot of commotion in the kitchen that woke me up around 11 p.m. Shuffle, shuffle. Faucet on, faucet off. Refrigerator opened, refrigerator closed. I don't think a drawer, cupboard, or counter top went untouched.

I thought it might be the Easter Bunny, but it would have been a day late for that. The results, however, were like an Easter egg hunt as Mother Dear moved things here, there, and just about everywhere.

The next morning, my first task was to inspect the garbage and recycle bins because one never knew what may have been deemed trash and treated as such. I attributed the loss of a box of tax preparation software to a prior reorganization of the den.

* * *

The lapse between the ability of someone to think of something, form the thought, and then put it into words causes gaps in the process of communication. A game of 20 (or more) questions ensues.

Mom appeared at the door to the home office as I clackety clacked on the computer keyboard and stared into the screen.

Mom: Would you help me with something?

Me: Sure, what can I do for you?

She stood holding a tissue.

Mom: Would you get me one of these?

I turned to the left in my chair, pulled another from the Kleenex box next to me on the desk, and handed it to her.

Me: There you go!

She took it and placed it on top of the one already in her hand. She left the room but came back shortly after.

Mom: Would you help me with something?

Me: Sure, what can I do for you?

Sound familiar? Yep, we hadn't reached the end of the game!

Mom: I want you to get me something.

Me: I got a tissue for you a little while ago. Is that what you're after?

She looked down at them in her hand. She was thinking and getting frustrated.

Mom: No. Dammit, I'm so stupid.

She touched her fingers to her mouth.

Me: Are you hungry? Do you want something to eat?

Sometimes she wanted me to pop the top on a can of soda or peel the foil off the top of a pudding cup.

Mom: No.

Me: Why don't you show me what you want since you can't say it and then I'll get it for you?

Mom: [Increasingly frustrated.] Oh, I don't know what I want.

I followed her out into the kitchen. Then she said it.

Mom: I just want to go out in the den, relax, and have a cigarette.

Me: Ohhhhhhh, you want a cigarette?

She looked down at her hand and held it out to show me the tissues again.

Mom: Yes! A cigarette!

Me: I'm sorry to disappoint you but we don't have any cigarettes in the house.

Mom: Oh, okay.

Mother Dear had smoked many years prior to this. When I was little, she smoked Newport's with the green colored packaging that denoted menthol. I remember her quitting cold turkey around 1970. She started up again in the mid-70s with Silva Thins and stopped again around 1980. Again, no slow reduction to wean herself off of her pack-a-day habit, she just stopped and didn't smoke again.

* * *

Mom summoned me into the bedroom because "there's a girl in there that I can't do anything with...she won't talk or anything." There was no girl and she was perplexed when I turned on the light and showed her no one was there. She pulled back the covers on the bed, expecting to catch the girl hiding, and still nothing. Neither of the two cats was there, either. Maybe she'd had a dream or noticed a change of lighting in the room? She shrugged her shoulders and I told her to go back to bed.

The event reminded me of a story that Grandma had told about Pop. My mother's father suffered from dementia and he got out of bed one morning at 4 a.m. and went to the window and kept yelling, "Be quiet! Would you be quiet?" He heard turkeys gobbling in the yard and they were disrupting his sleep. Except that the turkeys only existed in his mind, brought back to life from decades earlier.

That wasn't the only time Mom awoke, thinking someone was in the room.

Time: 4:32 a.m.

Mom: [Scared yelling.] Ahhhhhhhhhhhh! Ahhhhhhhhhhh!

I jumped up out of bed and ran to her.

Me: What's the matter?

Mom: He's gonna shoot me! HE'S GONNA SHOOT ME!

I looked around the room. Was I missing something?

Me: Who?

Mom: [Pointing at the empty chair.] HIM!

Me: There's no one here. You're okay. It was just a bad dream.

And back to bed I went.

———

Not too many nights later my sleep was interrupted again.

Time: 3:29 a.m.

Mom: [Yelling.] Noooooooooooo!

I woke up.

Mom: [Yelling.] Noooooooooooo!

I got up, rushed through the house, and into mother's bedroom.

Me: What's the matter?

Mom: He was on top of me!

I looked over and one of our cats was sitting on the nightstand. My best estimation of what had happened is that Mom combined a dream with Chiquita getting on her chest for some sleepy time. This wasn't usually a problem since they spent hours doing that every morning with Mom kissing, rubbing, and scratching the kitty.

Me: Don't worry. It was just a dream.

Mom: Don't act so innocent.

I returned to the couch and tried to get back to sleep.

Mother Dear came to wake me up. Poke. Poke. Poke. I came out of my unconsciousness. Mom was poking me on the hip. Poke. Poke. Poke.

The first time she had awoken me that night was because she thought one of the cats was dead. She was very upset. I got up and went into her bedroom to discover that, no, nothing was dead. This happened the next night as well. I figured out that she had mistaken a little stuffed panda bear for our black and white tuxedo cat. She woke up, looked at it, and it didn't move. She was too afraid to face the reality that her kitty might be dead.

Animals have always brought her such love and comfort. As she started to feel more and more helpless, the worry that she might lose them became a serious concern and high priority for her.

About 15 minutes later, she had time to reflect on what happened with the cat. She returned with a different story and she was even more upset. The "something's dead" feeling was still with her but this time she told me that *she* was dead. I comforted her, convincing her that it had all been a bad dream and led her through the house to show her that no one was in the house let alone anyone dead.

The story changed again upon my next awakening. I heard her shuffling in and stop by the side of the bed. When I opened my eyes, her hand was near my throat! For a split second, I thought she was trying to kill me, with all the talk about someone being dead!

She was checking to see if I was alive. She was having another "someone's dead" moment.

Me: What's the matter?

She continued to silently stare at me.

Me: Is there anything wrong?

She looks dazed and sat on the bed next to me. I'd been through this drill before.

Mom: Gavin is dead. [She started crying.]

Me: I'm Gavin and I'm talking to you so I'm not dead. You're talking to me so you're not dead either.

That was a little preemptive consoling to keep her from going there.

Mom: Well someone is dead.

Me: No, you've had this dream before. It's a bad dream but everything is okay. Now go back to bed.

She was in a cloudy world and she looked down at the floor as she tried to figure it out. After a few minutes, the fear of my death had left her and she got up and disappeared out into the kitchen. I rolled over and went back to sleep.

* * *

Late in the evening, around 8 p.m., Mom started asking when we were going home. I kept telling her that we *were* home but she would scoff. After about twenty times of repeating the conversation, she asked, "Why do you keep saying that?" I noted that what she said indicated that she did remember my previous responses even though her short-term memory was practically non-existent. Any rememberance was a good thing.

After several rounds of explaining that we were home with no success of convincing her, I decided to turn the tables.

Me: If we aren't home, then where is home? Describe to me where you want to go.

I figured I'd get some form of "the farm." Instead, I had thrown her for a loop. She was more confused than ever.

Mom: There's something really wrong.

I let it go at that and she dozed off. Then she was talking in her sleep.

Mom: My son is here and if I can't do it myself, I have to get him to help me.

Keen insight into what she was thinking. I'm not even sure she identified me as the son that she was speaking about. Yet she acknowledged that she couldn't do things and needed to reach out for help.

To someone with dementia, his or her thoughts and feelings, regardless of how impossible or improbable, are real. Their insecurities and confusion, from the events of the day or some form of occurrence in the past, are real.

* * *

I believe in karma. I also believe that the more self-aware you are, the quicker you realize when bad karma comes back to haunt you. Sometimes the karma is silly.

We had a futuristic "atomic clock" that synced up automatically with a satellite. Besides the time, it had the date, phases of the moon, and temperature inside the house, with a remote glued to the outside of the house that reported the temperature outside. When the batteries were replaced, it took a while for it to cycle and receive the time signal from outer space and reset the clock.

The clock's batteries had died so I replaced them. As I set the unit back on the shelf, the time was way off since it reset to 12:00 a.m.

Mom never knew what time it was, and she often got confused when the other clock in the room stopped running. It was a wonderful cuckoo clock brought back by a friend who had vacationed in the Bavarian Alps of Germany. Three metal pinecones suspended on chains ran the clock, the cuckoo, and four dancers that twirled every half hour. Sometimes Mom would look at the time displayed on the atomic clock when the pendulum on the cuckoo had stopped. It amused me to think about her looking at the atomic clock with its now-incorrect time.

Yet another clock, operated by battery power in the den where I slept, had been slowing down and I needed to replace its AA battery but hadn't. Remember I spoke about karma? That clock stopped the next morning at 7 a.m. When I woke up, I thought it was awfully light out to be so early in the morning. It was really 9:20. The joke was on me and it served me right for laughing to myself about Mom looking at the wrong time on the clock.

* * *

The sounds of summer's little buggers drove us nuts at night.

Quack, quack, quack, quack.

Quack, quack.

Quack, quack, quack, quack.

Mom: What's making that racket? They're driving me crazy!

Me: [*Thinking* to myself.] Umm, that train's already left the station.

I thought we were listening to tree frogs until I did some searching on the Internet and found the exact sound in a .wav file. The chirping came from Common True Katydids, relatives of grasshoppers and crickets, which are nearly flightless insects that inhabit the crowns of deciduous trees. They were hiding in the tops of our maple and birch trees.

Both male and female katydids make the 'quacking' sound by rubbing their front wings together and they listen for each other with ears located on their front legs. Breeding season is in late summer and early fall so that was the reason for the cacophony.

Over the years, I had systematically killed ground wasps that were burrowing in the front yard during their active phase in late June. Their food of choice? Katydids. And what happens when their natural enemy doesn't eat the katydids? They multiply and teach you a lesson by keeping you awake at night with their incessant, annoying mating calls.

* * *

My neighbors invited me next door for dinner. It was one of the few social engagements I could accept because I was able to keep an eye out for Mom from there. I didn't have to worry too much about her. The following day at lunch time, I was relating a conversation we had the previous night to my brother, and my mother was sitting in the chair listening to me re-tell the story. The neighbor's daughter had recently broken up with her boyfriend and he had contacted her a month later to retrieve some of his things, and I told them my philosophy on break ups.

Me: [To my brother, Mom listening.] I told them that leaving something behind is a classic ploy. When you break up with someone, you pack up all of their shit and mail it to them. That way you never have to see them again.

Mom: [To my brother.] That's what he's going to do to me.

She tipped her head in my direction, pursing her lips.

Me: [To Mom.] No! I wasn't talking about you. I was talking about the girl next door and how she shouldn't see her ex-boyfriend again or she'll get sucked back into a bad relationship.

Mom: [Looking away with a grimace.] Mmm-hmmm.

I'm not sure where that came from but you could see her demeanor change completely as soon as the idea of being placed in a facility crossed her mind. I wondered if all elderly folks were worried about being placed in assisted-care or a nursing home? Did this cross her mind often, or just when something was said that triggered it? Was she expressing fear that I was going to leave?

* * *

My Mom's brain combined facts from various events and created new "realities."

Example 1

The Real Reality

My father literally dropped dead of a massive heart attack in our backyard. My mother discovered him when she arrived home from work one afternoon and the neighbors called 911 when they figured out why she was screaming.

When the paramedics arrived, "Mr. June" showed up as part of the response team. Knowing that my father hated him, my Mom kept yelling to keep him away from the scene.

Months later, she bought an angel statue and put it in the yard under the 50' spruce trees where my father had been found.

About 20 yards away and years later, a stump in the backyard needed grinding and removal so my brother hired a crew of guys with a special machine to do the work. It was a rather big stump and Mom had insisted for years that someone was buried in the yard underneath it as if it was a cemetery headstone.

The crew arrived with a large machine with spinning blades that moved back and forth and were lowered just a bit with each pass. It ground away the stump and larger roots into small wood chips and sawdust.

Mom: It's about time someone got down here and helped me get out that stump. I was going at it with an axe just last night.

Mother's Reality

The stump was a burial marker and Mr. June was buried in the backyard under the tree stump. She had been trying to remove it by chopping at it with an axe.

Example 2

The Real Reality

Mom was on the side of the garage weeding the bed of irises and ended up fainting in the yard from the heat. That side of the house faced south and the white aluminum siding reflected the direct sun, making it particularly hot.

As part of my efforts to keep her from weeding again, I told her that I didn't want the neighbors to find her that way, sprawled out on the sidewalk. If she ever broke a hip, they would call 9-1-1 and she'd be in the hospital, which would be the beginning of the end. She tended to respond better if she thought people might disapprove of her. I thought a little scare might get through to her.

Mother's Reality

The neighbors are complaining that she doesn't take care of her yard so she thought she had to go out and work in the yard even more, exactly opposite of my intentions.

* * *

My brother told me that when he was alone with her, she always expressed concern about what was going to happen to her when I left.

Mom: If he moves back to California, it's gonna be awful lonely around here.

I wasn't moving back but there was worry in her statement. On some level, perhaps more than I realized, she knew the predicament we were in.

* * *

Mom woke up and called me into the bedroom with a weak and raspy voice.

Me: What's the matter?

Mom: I'm dying.

Me: What do you mean? What's wrong?

Mom: Something's not right.

Me: Do you feel sick? Do you hurt?

Mom: Yes. My neck hurts when I turn it. I think it's broken.

She had been sleeping with her head on two pillows and basically she had a crick in her neck. I removed the top pillow and she put her head down. Crisis averted!

* * *

Mom was talking to herself out in the kitchen. I was in the den working on the computer. She hollered to me seeking assistance with something.

Mom: Can you help me with these things?

I got up and headed out into the other room.

Me: Help you with what things?

Mom: Those things.

She pointed to our electric stove. The heating coils had been unplugged and removed, as well as the metal collector pans underneath them.

Me: Why did you remove them in the first place?

Mom: Because I'm an idiot.

Finding the humor in the most ridiculous of events that happen every day can help keep one's own sanity in the unpredictable and often ugly face of dementia.

PETS

The aquarium in the corner of the knotty pine-paneled breezeway, whether filled with salt or fresh water, was always active with brightly colored specimens. The filter, stuffed with a puff of fiberglass, kept the fish healthy and vibrant while it hummed away with comforting white noise. They swam through the ceramic castle nestled into the gravel on the bottom and avoided the periodic burst of bubbles slowly floating to the top from a nearby treasure chest.

Our home saw its share of pets over the years. Besides the rotation of angelfish and neon tetras, we had dogs, cats, turtles, a canary, and an orange and white guinea pig named Fluffy. The only thing missing was a partridge in a pear tree to complete the menagerie.

The cats were always allowed the run of the house, spending the bulk of their time outside during the summer and indoors during the winter. Kikky, the solid black kitten that my brother brought home from our school's summer recreation program, was originally called Spooky. I was young and said "Kikky" when I tried to say "Kitty," and it stuck.

She was an excellent predator, dropping mice, chipmunks, birds, and rabbits on the front stoop after her hunting expeditions were complete.

Kikky snuggled up against my mother and slept with her every night for over a decade, enjoying the winter months most when the gold electric blanket with satin edging was turned on. She favored lying on top of the firecracker-shaped connections where the lengths of the embedded wires were joined within the fabric. The heat was particularly intense there. More than being toasty, the cat's body temperature, fur, and the blanket itself escalated the temperature between the sheets to a practically unbearable level. Like demons from hell were throwing fireballs at the bed as they danced around the room.

We kept one of her three kittens, a black-and-white male named Muffin. He had a rough life, surviving the removal of a huge tumor from his stomach and having an eye poked out by a suspected blue jay. Once he'd been missing for several days when my mother heard him crying in the backyard. She found him under the hedgerow, clawing his way home with his front paws, dragging along his limp body with open wounds that were covered with maggots. His hind legs were damaged and his tail was broken when a car had hit him. If you could say that any cat had bad luck and the proverbial nine lives, he'd be the one.

He went missing one Thanksgiving and I searched for him before we left to spend the day with our relatives. I called out his name as I walked through the neighbors' yards and the fields behind the house. I checked the road to see if he hadn't survived another altercation with a vehicle. I looked and listened but we never saw him again. Did he wander off to die or did something else happen to him?

Kikky lived several years longer and died of old age. The loss of my father, her parents, and all of her pets left Mom very lonely. She was all alone in her empty nest.

Mom was terribly upset when Tasha our Alaskan Malamute had to be euthanized. Having her from a puppy, she became gravely sick at the age of 10. The diagnosis of heartworm didn't hold out much hope. Aegrescit medendo: the cure is sometimes worse than the disease. We began to give her arsenic pills, which were supposed to kill the parasite within. As her appetite waned, it became harder to get her to take the pills, even when concealed in roast beef.

The veterinarian said he would make a house call to put her to sleep in the afternoon. I spent the morning digging a grave in the backyard as the dog watched with woebegone eyes. She knew what was happening, I was sure of it. My father held the dog during the administration of the drug and buried her. I couldn't watch and went to work at my part-time job at the Grand Union grocery store about an hour later.

When Mother Dear got home and saw that the dog was no longer there, she began to cry hysterically. The tears and wails kept going until one point my father considered calling the rescue squad to calm her down from an anxiety attack.

She never spoke of the dog again.

Many years later, Whiskers moved in next door as an adoption from an animal shelter. She was a female cat who had lost one of her fangs from abuse and her black-and-white coloring was nearly identical to Muffin's tuxedo. Whiskers loved communing with nature, often spotted straddling the limb of a tree with her legs draped on either side to appreciate the cool breezes on hot and humid days.

If Whiskers were a person, she'd have been a gardener. Regardless of when Mother Dear set out to do yard work, Whiskers would show up to lend her supervision and companionship. She spent most of her afternoons with my mother, sitting in the grass like a regal sphinx with her front legs crossed, or snoozing under the lawn chair where Mom was laying to enjoy the sun and work on her tan.

When the same neighbors brought home a couple of high-energy Bishon Frise puppies, Whiskers spent less and less time at home, and more and more time with Mom, who became deeply attached. Mom began to let the cat in the house, feed her, and she eventually transitioned from living with her former owners to living with Mother. It seemed like a great solution because the neighbors knew that their dogs and the cat got along like, well, cats and dogs. They still saw the cat all the time; she just ate and slept somewhere else that provided a calmer environment.

The cat picked up a new name in addition to a new residence — Pooh Pooh. Paula called the cat a Godsend, arriving at the perfect time to lift my mother's spirits and give her unconditional love.

Her arrival, however, also brought worry. Mom became obsessed with the location of the cat. If she knew where the cat was, she could keep it safe. Unable to remember if the cat was inside or not, my brother made a sign that hung from the knob on the front door. "In" and "Out" were on opposite sides. Mom was to turn the sign when the cat entered or left. This gave her a way to keep track. It worked for a while until Mom forgot about the sign in addition to the cat's whereabouts.

Two years after my return home, we integrated a new cat into the household. Chiquita was so named because she was the runt of the litter and the Spanish term for "little one" was aptly chosen. It's a name we're all accustomed to with the brand of bananas, but Mom just couldn't master it, calling her Conchita instead. Cats rarely come when you call them so I'm not sure it really mattered.

Chiquita had a white moustache, bib, and boots, a soft gray coat, a short tail with faint rings, and malformed rear hip joints that caused an odd hopping gait when she was in a hurry. An even-tempered, friendly little cuss, she was a lap cat indoors that held on to Mom's knees with needle sharp claws that elicited an "Ouch!" at least once a sitting.

When outside, her personality set her on a mission to win the hearts and minds of the neighbors, visiting them all and quickly adding them to her list of friends.

Both Pooh Pooh and Chiquita were 12-year-old spayed females when they met. The first step was to keep the two separate within the house and slowly make them aware of each other. Chiquita was placed upstairs and kept inside while Pooh Pooh stayed on the main floor and was able to go out. I made them aware of each other by placing each on opposite sides of a door. They could smell each other and glimpse moving feet under the opening along the bottom. Slowly, I showed them to each other and then placed them in the same room together with my supervision.

When I was comfortable that Chiquita had adjusted to her new house, I walked around the yard several times as I held her, giving her a quick show of the property and how to find the door to come in. As expected, Pooh Pooh asserted her property rights and tried to establish the dominant role since she was the one with the homestead to defend. She was more aggressive and picked fights, but the tide turned as Chiquita became more familiar with her surroundings. Initially their altercations — generally restricted to growling, posturing, and slaps without claws extended — were related to Chiquita's mood. If she was relaxed and happy there weren't any problems, but if she was frisky then there was sure to be a dust up. Each of them was wary of passing the other for fear of attack. Their relationship reminded me of human sisters, or frenemies — friendly enemies. They liked each other when they weren't being competitive or adversarial.

As part of her routine, Pooh Pooh slept on top of Mom all night, would ask to be let out around 6 a.m. to patrol her territory and do her business, then came back inside about 8 a.m. for breakfast. That was up until the morning Chiquita decided to jump up on the bed. A squabble ensued directly on Mother Dear's chest complete with hissing, growling, and screaming (that was Mom). Pooh Pooh wound up with a bloody nose from a scratch and my mother just about had a heart attack. Pooh Pooh lost the battle and the war, never sleeping with my mother again, supplanted by Chiquita who claimed the sleeping spot as her own.

The cats occupied so much of my mother's time. It was a blessing because I would have been the constant center of attention and a raving lunatic without them. It was bad enough with them around. Mom wondered where they were or if they were hungry. It gave her purpose. The cats did love her and shared turns on her lap getting petted, scratched, hugged, and kissed.

To say that the cats were spoiled would be an understatement. They meowed, "Jump" and we asked, "How high?"

Still, there was plenty of time for some lighthearted teasing. Chiquita was in the den with Mom and me. We were sitting on the couch and the cat was sitting in the center of a dark green Native American patterned area rug on the floor in front of us. Along the back of the couch were two large members of Mom's stuffed teddy bear collection — a standard brown type and a panda.

I grabbed the brown bear and held him so he appeared to be standing on the floor facing the cat. Chiquita's eyes started to get big and her pupils dilated black. I rocked the bear back and forth pretending that it was walking towards her. With no warning, she jumped about a foot in the air, ran through the house at breakneck speed, and then up the stairs to hide under a bed. Mom and I laughed the hardest we had in a long time and it gave us some much-needed comic relief.

Poor thing. I had no idea it would scare her so. It took the cat two days to get up the courage to go back in that room.

* * *

Share and share alike was Mom's attitude regarding the cats. One morning I found some pumpkin pie in the cats' food dishes and another time they were served orange-flavored soda in their water bowl. There were times that the dementia caused her to do odd things because she didn't understand the items, and other times there were miscues because a lack of memory was at play.

I found Mom eating mini Reese's peanut butter cups in the kitchen and I noticed there was white stuff in the cat's dish on the floor at her feet. I asked her about it but she seemed puzzled. She had opened a carton of ice cream and spooned a scoop into the cat dish. She had forgotten she was getting it for herself when her attention was diverted to the candy. I dished up a new bowl for her and got her situated back on the couch watching television.

I had prepared a nice tenderloin roast for dinner. Mom hadn't been very interested in beef for a long time. I liked it, and she'd eat it on occasion, so I'd make it to break up the monotony of chicken. I sliced the beef into bite size pieces so she didn't have to worry about cutting it. It was a very tender piece of meat that was easy for her to chew. As the side dish, I put a couple spoonfuls of macaroni salad on her plate.

I served the meal to her in the breezeway where we could watch television. A few minutes had passed when I heard the odd sounds of eating. It wasn't Mom. I looked over and Chiquita was sitting on the sofa next to her licking the mayonnaise off of the elbow noodles. Mom continued to spear the meat with her fork as she watched the cat sharing her food.

Me: Mom, don't let the cat eat off your plate!

Mom: But she's obviously hungry.

I couldn't argue with that and I had to appreciate when she actually put forth a logical argument. The cat hopped down when she was done, licking the sides of her paws and rubbing them against her cheeks and whiskers to clean her face. Mom smiled and everyone was happy.

That is, until I heard the sound of a fork scraping across a plate. Mom had the plate back on her lap and was moving the remainder of the salad into a small heap. Then, without thinking, she scooped a fork full of salad and moved it towards her open mouth. It seemed like it was happening in slow motion.

Me: [Shouting.] Don't eat that!

Mom: [Jumping and startled.] Why not?

She was perturbed.

Me: [Scowling.] Because the cat's been licking on it.

I'm very particular when it comes to the cleanliness of pets. Cats are relatively clean but I always wash my hands after petting them. I generally don't pet dogs unless they're mine and I wash my hands thoroughly afterwards. When I see people give their pets a lick of an ice cream cone and then return to eating it themselves? I gag and make a mental note never to eat at their house. Ever. From then on, everything they prepare becomes suspect.

I've heard the argument that a dog's mouth is cleaner than a human's. I don't believe it, and even if I did, I wouldn't care. Pets are not human. It's safe to say that most humans don't lick their privates just before slobbering on a scoop of Cherry Garcia. And if they did, they wouldn't get any of my ice cream, either.

Mom: What are you talking about?

Me: Don't you remember that the cat was just licking the food on your plate?

Of course she didn't remember and shook her head like I was crazy. I took her plate out to the kitchen where I promptly disposed of what was left.

* * *

Our location in suburbia provided a great vantage point to enjoy the active wildlife. The bird feeders, hung on hooks from the eaves, dangled a foot in front of the windows. They hosted cardinals, tufted titmice, goldfinches, chickadees, starlings, juncos, and sparrows. I made suet of lard, crunchy peanut butter, wheat germ, oatmeal, corn meal, and flaxseeds that attracted every type of woodpecker native to the area — downy, hairy, red-breasted, and pileated.

We watched three wild tom turkeys wander through the field behind the house. Pooh Pooh was outside by the shed watching, too. The cat crouched on top of the snow, which had formed a hard crust after some misting rain and freezing temperatures a few days before. The fowl strutted their way across the yard in a pecking parade then disappeared into the weeds.

The following day several deer meandered along the same path. Remembering that the cat had been out in the field before, Mom started to worry. I tried to assuage her fears.

Me: The cats go out all the time. They know about the deer. Why are you so worried?

Mom: Because deer will maul a cat!

That would be a heck of a sight, although I'm not sure there's any record of a cat being mauled by a deer. The cats wouldn't take on the squirrels, possums, or skunks in the backyard because they were too big. I couldn't imagine them getting very close to a deer.

* * *

Mom began to insist that we had three cats. She was always doing a head count on where all the cats were and she could never find the third. When I asked her what its name was or what it looked like, she didn't know. She just insisted we had three.

On my computer desk, I kept a large photo of the cat that I had for 16 years. He was a beautiful Abyssinian, full of personality, and she had met him on visits to see me in California. She looked at the picture and asked me to remind her of his name. I prompted her that his name was Solomon and then it dawned on me...he (via his picture) was the missing third cat!

Solomon had been a handful and a half, and I loved him every day of the time I had him. When he was naughty, I'd chastise him, telling him, "You deserve to be spanked!" He was never hit — he was way too pampered for that. I'd wag my finger at him, just to let him know that jumping up onto the counter or any other disciplinary infraction he'd just committed was not going to be tolerated. Until the next time he did it, of course.

He would look up at me with a disbelieving face when I gave him such a stern warning. Often I'd tell him, "Because you're so evil. You were born that way!" I'd say these things in a normal tone of voice so the cat wasn't being yelled at; he just thought I was talking to him about some nonsense in the same language that Charlie Brown's teacher uses.

I'd say odd, terrible things to the pets because I found it so funny and they had no idea what I was saying anyway. The more outrageous, the better, as far as I was concerned!

When Pooh Pooh and Chiquita spent most of their time inside for weeks at a stretch during the cold months, they would put on some extra winter weight, getting chubby bellies with less exercise.

Me: [Referring to Chiquita.] We're gonna have that little butterball for dinner tomorrow. I'll put an apple in her mouth just like they do in China!

Mom: Why would you say such a thing?

She had a grin on her face so I thought she was playing along. I thought it was pretty clear that I had no intention of eating the cat for dinner regardless of what they do in China or how tasty a roasted apple might be.

Me: Because she was born bad, and it's been downhill ever since.

Mom's eyes pleaded for some reassurance. Then the water works started. She was crying. Real tears. That's when it dawned on me that she wasn't in on the joke at all and thought I was serious. I quickly set the record straight but the fun was lost on her.

I changed the subject, it was quickly forgotten, and the cat won a stay of execution and wouldn't be on the dinner table after all.

* * *

Her love for pets and her inability to make sound judgments proved to be a dangerous mix.

One day she was doing yard work by keeping up with the leaves being shed by our maple trees. Having a nice yard was an obsession for her and the Alzheimer's hadn't changed that a bit. It was beneficial, giving her the chance to get out of the house for some fresh air, to enjoy the yard, and get a bit of exercise.

It was a gorgeous autumn day and Pooh Pooh was sitting in the middle of the street in front of the house. Our dead end road didn't carry much traffic and the kitty was street smart. A car came down the road and the cat headed for the neighboring yard to get out of the way. Mother Dear darted out into the road shouting, "Save the cat!" The car saw both of them and went slowly so there was no danger of either getting hit.

It all happened so quickly. Just when you think all is safe, something unexpected can happen.

Putting herself in harms way to protect an animal is what she would do. The alternative of losing a pet would be far worse for her than any injury to herself.

LOST

I heard her say, "I'm lost."

I had been asleep (it was 6:15 a.m.) and she was standing in the middle of the room. I looked at her and she seemed almost in fear, but too confused to let that emotion sink in.

I got up and explained where she was. The two cats were awake and watching the whole thing. I pointed to them, which was always a good way to get Mom to snap back into some form of normalcy.

Me: The kitty cats are here.

Mom: I have to go to the bathroom.

She had a look on her face like she was going to go right then and there. I acted quickly and got her into the bathroom. I waited for her outside the closed door and then lead her to back to bed when she was done.

Best I could tell, she had gotten up to go to the bathroom and had forgotten where she was and what she was doing. I thought the day was going to be a rough one. But, surprisingly, it wasn't. She called me into the bedroom about 10 a.m. to show me that Chiquita was laying on her chest, under the covers, with both of their heads the only thing visible.

It's a strange disease!

* * *

When Mom "wandered" for the first time it began a new dimension to the disease. Many Alzheimer's patients develop a behavior of wandering and then getting lost. When they don't know where they are, or think they need to get home, they just start walking with no real end point. Worse, they could have access to a car and start driving. The further they go, the more lost they get.

That morning Mom seemed upset when the housekeeper was cleaning. She was agitated but I wasn't sure why. When I questioned her, she ignored me (no wonder I choose partners that are passive aggressive), put on a sweatshirt and jacket, and out the door she went.

We lived on a dead end street and she walked down towards the closed cul-de-sac. It was quite a ways to the end, maybe a tenth of a mile. At the end, a loop of pavement went around a fire hydrant with a tall red metal flag attached for visibility during snowy winters. I stood out of sight and watched her to see where she was going and to make sure nothing happened. She walked down the road, stopping every now and then to observe the various houses and yards, made the loop, and returned home.

She came in the house and after that she was in a good mood. Regardless of her safe return, leaving the house on an aimless mission was not a good sign.

* * *

I heard the front door open and saw Mother Dear pass the window as she headed down the sidewalk. It was only a few seconds earlier that she'd been sitting in the chair next to me. We had been watching the television in the front room when she got up and went through the archway out into the kitchen. She made her way through the house without saying a word and out the door she went.

I thought that she might have been headed out to pick up the mail or the newspaper at the end of our fairly long paved driveway since she could have seen the delivery boxes for each from her previous vantage point in the house. I later ascertained that she thought a sand covered clump of snow along the road was an injured or dead dog that needed rescue.

The dementia caused her to see a lot of things that she determined to be dead animals. I shouldn't say that all the imaginary animals she saw were dead when, in fact, she thought that many of the things she envisioned were actually alive.

As she headed across the street, not stopping at the mailbox, I hastily grabbed my coat, put on my shoes and hat, and ran out the door. It was 30°F outside and she was on a mission in the freezing cold without a jacket on.

She crossed the street without looking in either direction. Luckily there wasn't any traffic on the road. I finally caught up to her walking down the street after she'd investigated the lump and verified that there was no animal to be found.

Me: Where are you going?

Mom: Oh, around.

She swept her hand around as if she was a model on *The Price Is Right* showing off a spectacular new car.

Me: It's cold out here! You need to get inside or you'll freeze.

Mom: Yes, it is cold out here. Brrrrr.

She made her teeth chatter. That was a behavior I understood as a signal to demonstrate that she was cold when the words to explain it wouldn't come to her. She quickly reassessed her situation, determined that going home was the best course of action and started to walk up the next-door neighbor's driveway. Right idea, wrong house.

Me: That's not our house. Come on, we live next door. [I pointed to our house.]

Mom: That's not our house.

Me: [I pointed to the driveway.] Sure, don't you remember your red car and how the house has blue-painted accents?

Mom: That isn't blue, it's gray.

Me: Okay, our house is the one with the gray accents.

This seemed to satisfy her and we made it up our driveway and into the house. Going with the flow, instead of arguing to prove that you are right, is the path of least resistance in these situations. It's not about being right; it's about obtaining your objectives.

How easily that she could have died from exposure if no one had been around to monitor her. Outside in the cold, not knowing how to get home even though her house was right in front of her — she'd lived there for over 50 years.

* * *

Most of the frustration I felt, some days unbearable, was my mother's insistence on doing yard work. I'd have to worry about her overdoing it, feeling sick and wiped out the next day, or wandering off. It wasn't unusual to find her cleaning up the neighbor's yards. It was enough to make me dread the nice weather.

It had become a tiring battle that just wore me out. You can't use rational explanations with a person that thinks irrationally. And they don't ever tire of arguing because each time they start a tiff it's a brand new experience for them.

My first inclination to keep her safe was to erect a fence around the perimeter of the property to minimize the chance of any accidents during a wandering incident. It would provide her with a sense of freedom by allowing her access to the yard and permit her to enjoy the gardens — while keeping her from leaving and getting lost. I penciled out the costs, however, and it seemed a bit extreme and expensive.

Well, I found an answer. I present to you the swing! A few days later I discovered a porch swing in a Sunday newspaper circular and the simplicity of the solution was perfect. She enjoyed watching the hummingbirds drink the sugar-water 'nectar' from the bright red feeders with simulated plastic yellow flowers. She'd listen to the house wrens chatter as they built nests in each of the houses attached to the wrought iron trellis, and admired the landscaping filled with black-eyed Susans, daisies, irises, and a wide variety of hostas. Combine all that with frequent naps and it would keep her busy the entire summer. Problem solved with a better, more enjoyable, and less expensive solution!

This swing, $200 at Kmart and about three hours to assemble, was worth every penny and drop of sweat. Mom sat in the swing and rocked for two to three hours at a time. Even my brother couldn't believe she didn't hop up and start picking up leaves or pulling up weeds. This kept her in one place so I didn't have to worry about her wandering off.

I also discovered a nice little trick on the weeding. Get rid of the weeds. How did I do that without pulling them myself? I put down a black fabric barrier in most of the flowerbeds and covered it with pea gravel. Voila, a 90% reduction in weeding!

This made life immeasurably better for me and I think she enjoyed herself more, too. Pooh Pooh spent the better part of her day asleep on the swing and was a great companion for Mom as the two rocked the afternoons away.

Between downpours of rain, Mom made her way out into the back yard to rock on the swing. She was a bit like the Pied Piper as both cats always came to lie on the patio with her. You could never see them but they appeared out of nowhere as if they had been waiting for her to arrive.

I was working on the computer, but I'd get up to check on her about every 5-10 minutes. I knew she'd stay there a while once she got situated.

After about an hour, I heard her coming in the garage door and she made her way through the house to the back room where I was sitting. I looked up and she was upset.

Mom: I didn't know where I was. I didn't know how I got here or how I'm getting home.

She'd been crying but was okay when she started talking to me. I brought her back outside, sat on the swing with her, and explained where she was and that she owned this house. She couldn't get it through her head. We went over it and over it. When she was on the swing, she thought she was back at the camp on Babcock Lake, causing her disorientation.

* * *

After Mom started wandering, I began to consider all the options. With the loss of short-term memory comes unfamiliarity with their current location. Imagine if you woke up and didn't know where you were, who the people were that surrounded you, and all the sights and sounds were strange. The feeling of being lost, often frightened, could lead you to seek a place where you knew the environment and belonged.

It's this quest for the familiar that inspires them to leave where they are in search of where they think they should be. There is no plan when they go, no knowledge of how to get where they're headed. They are incapable of forming a plan. Their final destination may be in another state and/or not even exist at all anymore. Once they set out on their journey, they quickly become lost.

This change of behavior is also a turning point for care. The patient must be monitored around-the-clock. Time of day or even time of year is of no concern to them.

The strains on the caregiver increase exponentially because the ability to get a reprieve from the situation becomes increasingly limited with the constant care required.

* * *

While the swing was an excellent idea for the summer, it wasn't going to work in the cold and snowy winter. The swing would be put in the basement so another means of keeping Mom occupied was needed. Experience had shown that I couldn't rely on snow and freezing temperatures to be a fool-proof deterrent to her wandering.

Solutions come from odd places if you keep your mind open. I was on the phone with my best friend and I heard door chimes in the background. When I asked, Jennifer explained that they were part of her home's security system. Each door emitted a beeping sound when it was opened. If it worked to keep people out, I thought, it could work to keep people in!

An added bonus was that I would be able to sleep more soundly. I had been keeping one eye open in case she ventured out in the middle of the night. Mom was up a lot in the early morning hours so I could never be sure she wouldn't head out the door at 3 a.m. without me knowing it. There were times when she would come into the room where I was sleeping to tell me she didn't know where she was and what she was supposed to do. I would guide her into the bedroom, assure her everything was fine, and that it was time for her to go to sleep. Rather than waking me, she could have easily wandered out the door at the other end of the house and I'd have been none the wiser.

My quest for electronic door alerts began at a local department store. Nothing there, I discovered, although I was directed to the "child-proofing your home" area. That was a step in the right direction even though there wasn't anything in the way of door alarms. Next were trips to the local home improvement chains. One didn't have anything to offer in the store but an employee suggested that I place a special order for a device that would cost approximately $60 per unit. That would be $180 since there were three doors to be alarmed.

That was too expensive so I decided to look online. I've learned that the art of surfing the web is to start at a certain point and then follow leads that present alternatives that hadn't been considered.

Lo and behold, I found exactly what I was looking for at the bargain price of two for $10! The items were the Window or Door Alarm with entry chime mode from General Electric. They had two pieces, one that attached to the frame of the door and the other to the door itself. If the sensors in each piece became separated when the door was opened, a loud "Bing Bong" alarm was sounded. Escaping thwarted and peace of mind restored!

* * *

I was dozing on the couch and Mom was talking to the cat. I caught some of what she was saying, but since I wasn't really conscious, I heard some but missed most of it.

Mom: "I don't know who I am."

She'd been struggling the prior few days as to *where* she was but I never thought she didn't know *who* she was. It was a fine line when she made statements or asked questions like this. When you explained she usually got frustrated because she knew she was losing her mind. Most times, I ignored her and only got into a more complete explanation if she started a conversation about it. It seemed to be less upsetting if I just let it go. I didn't acknowledge the comment and pretended I was asleep.

TELEVISION

Watching the moon landing is one of my earliest memories. Hard to believe it was over 40 years ago in July of 1969. I was five years old, going on six, and my whole family was watching the color television in the breezeway.

"Come here, come here," they all shouted to me. "This is something you'll remember for the rest of your life!"

I ran out from the kitchen and sat on the cold white-tiled floor about three feet in front of the set, a large wooden console filled with tubes, fuses, and wires, and watched as the lunar module descended. The transmission showed the surface of the moon getting closer and closer. The spacecraft was slowly floating downward and beeping along the way.

When they touched down, my family cheered! This was one of life's historic moments that people remember exactly where they were when it happened.

While the television can bring triumph into our homes, it can also bring tragedy.

On the evening of Saturday August 30, 1997, I was working on the computer with CNN tuned on the television. In the background I heard the announcement. It didn't make sense. It was Princess Diana. She was in critical condition after a car accident in Paris. It was in a tunnel. There were paparazzi chasing her on motorcycles.

Was she with Dodi? Dodi was dead according to some reports. There was a swirl of information bits, as the newscasters were trying to put it all together as was I. She wasn't wearing her seat belt. Her bodyguard was alive. I watched "the crawl" along the bottom of the screen. Her condition changed from critical to grave. The only rating worse was dead. I was sick to my stomach. I had to escape.

I took off out of my apartment and my eyes were welling with tears. My mind was working feverishly. If I walked around the lake, a 20-30 minute outing depending on my pace, things would be better when I returned. The news anchors would have discovered an error in reporting or that it was a hoax of some sort. It was a walk that I made nearly every day for exercise and always made an extra lap when I was under stress and needed to clear my head.

It was so like me — check out for a bit and rely on the universe to make things right. If there were a Chinese astrology sign for an ostrich I would surely be it. As it was, I'm a rabbit and running away in the face of danger seemed to be in my cosmic makeup if not my DNA. Alas, it seemed the universe never came to my rescue.

If nothing else, the fresh air, tranquility, and manicured landscaping that the City of Irvine, CA provided would manage to calm me. When I returned I was sure the news would be more complete. They'd know the whole story. I knew she'd be fine. How could she be anything else? She was Diana.

My cat Solomon, my little buddy that always met me at the door, greeted me upon my return. We had a routine, he and I. When he heard my foot falls on the stairs and landing outside he raced to the door. I knew he was there on the other side of the door from his cries. Because he was an Abyssinian, he was a talker. I asked him repeatedly through the door, "Is there a little boy in this house?" He dutifully answered, "Meow!" He was so darn cute. I opened the door, so glad to see him. He stood squarely in front of me and looked up, which was his signal to be picked up. I obliged, gave him a kiss on the forehead, and made my way to the television. I had left it on in my haste to leave. I asked my kitty if Diana was okay. He didn't answer. But the news crawl had changed.

"PRINCESS DIANA HAS DIED IN PARIS"

I was sick. My stomach was in a knot. I wanted to cry. At the same time, I didn't want to cry. I was a man. What the hell was I thinking?

More news. Cameramen being held by Paris police in a van. My head was swimming. I held the cat tight. I thought about my upcoming trip to London. What did this mean? I was drawn back to the television, like watching a train wreck. Only worse. I knew her...

* * *

I tried to put on television programs that didn't have a plot because Mom wasn't able to follow any other types of shows. Reality programs, game shows, talk shows, sports, and the news fit her mental capabilities pretty well.

I had been a fan of *American Idol* from the beginning and it was a perfect formula that was easy to understand. Except Mom couldn't stand it when the judges criticized the talent.

> **Mom:** [About Randy Jackson.] Who the hell does he think he is?
>
> **Mom:** [About Simon Cowell.] Oh, there's that asshole. I can't stand that guy!

Simon was his normal acerbic self and made some particularly disparaging comments about one of the contestants. Mother Dear started booing, hissing, and yelling at him. It was like watching two shows in one and I wasn't sure which was more entertaining!

* * *

Mom became increasingly confused between reality and what was happening on television. There were times where she understood that these were television shows with actors. Other times it was as if she were watching real people and stories unfolding on television. Yet another take, was that these people were actually in the room interacting directly with her. Her reaction to the people on television was a good indication on what her mental status was at the moment.

On the one hand, her lack of knowledge and understanding was tragic while on the other hand her innocence was very captivating.

Science fiction presented the largest gap between what is obviously fiction and what is real.

Saturday and Sunday evenings were a funny night for watching television. I'm a *Star Trek* fan and enjoy watching any and all old episodes of the first series and the follow up *Star Trek: The Next Generation*.

A particular episode from the original series, *The Man Trap*, was a favorite of mine that pitted the crew of the USS Enterprise (NCC-1701) against a shape-shifting alien in dire need of salt to live. When it appeared as a human, it took the form of Nancy, an old flame of Dr. McCoy. This personal history gave him a vested interest in defending the villain since it only presented itself to him as his lost love. As its true incarnation, it was a hideously hairy beast with suction cups on its hands that drew all of the salt out of humans as nourishment for its own survival. It had killed several crewmembers, leaving strange red rings on their faces. The monster's true appearance was revealed to Dr. McCoy at the end of the episode when he, in shock, didn't know whether to save Captain Kirk or Nancy's alter ego. Thankfully Spock killed the sodium hungry murderer.

The final scene showed the spaceship Enterprise in orbit over an orange planet below.

Mom: I don't know what the hell kind of joint this is with crazy people flying around the universe.

Mom knew that this was supposed to be taking place in outer space. Did she think that space travel and alien beings were real?

About the same time there was a television commercial featuring Godzilla. Not a high-tech CGI monster, but a man in a cheesy monster suit stomping through a "city" that had been constructed to size like those used in the old-school films from Japan.

Mom: I wonder if things like that really exist?

Perhaps that answered the question of her belief in space travel and aliens beings.

* * *

I was in the living room and I had left Mom asleep in the den in front of the television. She awoke and was ready for bed. She always tried to turn off the television but couldn't figure out how to use the remote control. Sometimes she would get lucky and hit the power button.

I heard the television go off and within a couple of minutes, Mom was behind me asking for my help to shut things down. I turned and she was holding the remote control with a baffled look on her face.

I explained that the television was off and assured her that everything was ready for her to go to bed. She was insistent and growing impatient, so I followed her out to the other room. She was trying to turn off the porch lights using the remote control.

The following night I went to bed and left her awake in front of the

TV. The remote control was on the tray table in front of her.

In the morning, I found the remote and portable phone on the kitchen counter and the television was off. I went into the den and hit the power button on the remote to turn the television on. Nothing. I pressed it harder. Again, nothing. I thought I'd move closer and directly in front of the set and tried again in case the batteries' charge was low. Still nothing. I hit the button on the front of the TV and there was no response.

Well, Mother must not have had any success turning the television off with the remote because she'd unplugged it from the wall. Mission accomplished. While she couldn't figure out the remote, I noted that she understood that the television ran on electricity and unplugging it was a way to turn it off.

* * *

Mother Dear, my brother and I were sitting in the den. The television was off and Mom was sitting in a chair directly across from it.

Mom: Who's that in there?

Brother: Where?

Mom: [Pointing at the television.] In there!

My brother caught on before I did. She was looking at our reflections in the glass screen.

Brother: It's you.

Mom: What do you mean 'it's me'?

Brother: Do you think you can go in there and join them?

Me: You'd be like Alice in Wonderland going through the looking glass!

Brother: [Waving at the television.] Wave to them.

Mom waved, saw herself, and just wasn't putting two and two together.

Brother: See? It was you all along.

Mom finally figured it out and we all had a good laugh.

* * *

The perception of interacting directly with television personalities came most frequently during the local news programs. She was certain that newscasters and weather reporters in a close-up shot were in the room, looking at her, and speaking directly to her. She often responded to them with affirmations such as "Yup" and "Uh-huh" when they made a statement or posed a rhetorical question.

Mom had a bit of a paranoia streak in her. If anyone implied that she was the cause of something, no matter how inconsequential, she thought you were picking on her.

For instance, she frequently had sores on her nose and forehead. They started with a bit of dry skin and then she would scratch and pick at them until they turned into a sore. Telling her to stop when she was picking made her angry.

Mom: How come I have these sores on my face?

Me: Because you scratch at them when you aren't thinking about it.

Mom: [Angry.] Why is everything always my fault?

It didn't take too many times for this to happen in order for me to learn that the best response was to shrug my shoulders when she asked. When the spots got really irritated, I simply put Neosporin anti-bacterial ointment on them and covered them up with a Band-Aid. That helped them heal while preventing her from making them any worse.

But that isn't the story I planned on telling here. You just have to know that her mind-set was such that she often felt blamed.

We were watching a professional NBA basketball game on television. I'm a huge fan and Mom liked it, too. It went back decades when she had a crush on Los Angeles Lakers guard Jerry West after whom the NBA logo is designed.

After a controversial play involving a foul called on one of his players, coach Rick Adelman leaped from the bench and started yelling at the referees.

Mom: Oooo, he's mad.

Adelman turned and it appeared as though he was looking right into the camera and shouting. We had upgraded to a rather large 42" high-definition flat panel screen and Mother Dear thought he was looking directly at her and going to blame her for why he was angry.

Mom: [Defensively, to avoid blame.] Don't look at me!

* * *

In other sports news, we were watching the U.S. Open tennis tournament. At the time, we were under the threat of Hurricane Hanna marching up the east coast of the U.S. and dumping a lot of rain on us.

For some reason, it was raining here in upstate NY but not Flushing Meadows where the tournament was being played. Odd because they were south of us and should have experienced the rain first.

Anyway, it was raining outside but not in New York City or on the television where play continued.

Mom: How come they keep playing in the rain?

Me: Well it's raining here but it isn't raining there.

Mom: Where are they?

Me: Down in New York City.

Mom: Oh.

I think it registered on some level because she seemed satisfied by my answer. I'm still not sure she understood how it could be raining here and not there on the television at the same time, since the television itself was here where it was raining.

* * *

People who suffer from dementia often get off schedule regarding days and nights. The shorter days in the winter seem to exacerbate the problem. There were periods of time, weeks perhaps, that Mom would be up most of the night and sleep until noon.

I thought Mom's nighttime escapades were related to symptoms of sundowning. Sundown syndrome is an observed behavior that many Alzheimer's patients have that causes an odd state of confusion when the sun begins to go down. Borrowing from WebMD.com:

> *Sundowning, or sundown syndrome, affects some people who have Alzheimer's disease and dementia. People with dementia who "sundown" experience periods of increased confusion and agitation as the sun goes down — and sometimes through the night.*
>
> *Sundowning may prevent people with dementia from sleeping well. It may also make them more likely to wander. Sundowning is a common cause of caregiver burnout.*

Here in the northeastern U.S., it gets dark about 4 o'clock in the winter months and about 9 p.m. in the summer. The script of Mom's episodes of disorientation revolved around who owned the house, where she was, that she needed to go home, etc.

I had cut back on her brain chemistry drugs in order to give the new Alzheimer's medications, Aricept and Namenda, a chance to work with a minimum of competing drug effects. Both of these drugs were supposed to be effective and, when used together in combination, had results greater than the sum of each if used separately.

If Mom didn't show any improvement, I wanted to be able to say that the drugs didn't work rather than a complication from interacting with her Paxil (depression) and Xanax (anxiety) meds. She tolerated the Aricept and Namenda fine although there wasn't much improvement in memory. We decided, with her doctor's approval, to keep her on them in an effort to prevent any further memory loss even if she wasn't realizing any improvement in capabilities.

I would try to give her subtle cues that it was time to go to bed.

Me: Well, it's beddie-bye time. I'm going in to sleep.

That usually didn't work and she would keep staring into the television. With 24-hour cable, there's always something on. I considered getting a little more forceful in my approach but, honestly, it was a hassle that I just as soon not get tangled up in. Caregivers learn to pick their battles to conserve their energy.

Me: It's time for bed. Are you coming?

Mom: Well, I suppose I should, too.

I turned off the television and started in to bed. She got up, got her drinking glass and put it in the kitchen sink, and started in after me. I hopped on the couch in the den, covered up with an afghan, and closed my eyes.

Bing! I heard the TV pop back on in the other room. She didn't seem able to figure out how to use the remote, but when push came to shove, sometimes she managed. Perhaps she got lucky by pushing every button there was until something happened. As my uncle always said, "Even a blind squirrel finds a nut once in a while!"

* * *

We were watching *The 101 Most Unforgettable SNL Moments* (Saturday Night Live) on the *E!* cable channel.

Steve Martin and Dan Aykroyd: We are two wild...

Mom: ...and crazy guys!

It's amazing that many of these catch phrases are so deeply embedded in the American lexicon that someone with Alzheimer's can still quote them generations later.

* * *

We would watch reruns of *Jeopardy!* during lunch. I'm quite good at it and Mom always smiled at me when I got the correct answer. "You should be on there," she'd say. Except I knew I'd pull a Cindy Brady and stare blankly in sheer terror when the little red light on top of the camera came on.

Alex Trebek: This river and its tributaries drain most of South America.

Mom: Amazon.

Contestant: What is the Amazon?

Alex: Correct. Select again.

Mom: I said that.

Mother wasn't beyond answering a few, much to my amazement.

* * *

Just when I thought she believed everything she saw was actually happening, she recognized television sitcoms weren't real. When there was a funny scene on *I Love Lucy*, she asked:

Mom: How do they keep a straight face?

* * *

Mom was obsessed with two shows and she asked constantly when they'd be on. All day, every day, she asked, "Are my programs on today?"

She had ditched *The Young and The Restless* because she couldn't follow the complex story lines and multiple characters, in favor of *The Dr. Phil Show* and *Deal Or No Deal*. Dr. Phil was pretty easy for me to handle since it was on every day except the weekends. "It'll be on this afternoon" or "tomorrow afternoon" was an answer that satisfied her. She liked his no nonsense homespun advice and good old boy, aw shucks Texan personality.

It was more difficult with *Deal Or No Deal* because it was only on once a week. What's more, she couldn't understand the concept of the show because it was counterintuitive. Contestants selected one of 25 suitcases, each of which contained a dollar amount between $1 and $1,000,000. The contestant hoped they had selected the million. They tried to determine what was in their case by choosing from the remaining 24, one at a time, to reveal their contents and use a process of elimination. Periodically, they stopped the selection process and offered the contestant an odds-calculated set amount of money to hedge their bets and leave the show with a guaranteed amount. They could take the money and walk away or take their chances and keep going. The offered amount started out low and gradually got higher depending on what amounts had been revealed. For instance, if the million-dollar case was revealed, which meant the contestant didn't have it, then the offered amount didn't have to be as high to pursuade them to walk away.

Therefore, rather than getting excited about revealing high amounts, contestants were happy about picking low amounts because that meant their case had a better chance of containing a higher amount. Got that? Mom just couldn't understand why they would cheer for low amounts and get depressed when they revealed the $1M or other high amount. She probably asked 10 times during each show for me to explain it, and I'd patiently tell her every time. She thought selecting the million dollars was a good thing, not understanding that it wasn't what the contestant actually won.

The excitement of the show seemed to be the draw for her. Oh, and I think she had a bit of a crush on the host Howie Mandel, referring to him as "my guy."

* * *

Here in the Unites States, there is a company called GEICO Insurance that sells coverage for car, home, etc. They rely heavily on advertising to get business because of their direct sales model. The fact that they are a division of Warren Buffet's huge conglomerate Berkshire Hathaway means they have deep pockets for several different television ad campaigns that blanket the airwaves.

One features cavemen and the tagline, "So easy a caveman can do it," describing how easy it would be to switch insurance carriers. There was the initial commercial that used the concept, which spawned a whole slew of additional spots and a television show. The cavemen appear indignant and complain how they are being publicly humiliated and maligned because they are different from everyone else. They are portrayed as everyday people that do everyday things, with ordinary intelligence —they just happen to be cavemen. It's quite clever and amusing.

Every time one of these commercials came, Mom always said, "There's that guy again." She believed he really was a caveman!

Mom: You'd think he'd get a decent haircut.

There must be something about the advertising folks for GEICO. Mom continued to be absolutely enamored with the cavemen. If old ladies with dementia were their target market, they were hitting a bull's eye.

Another of their simultaneous ad campaigns featured a CGI-generated gecko character that played off of the GEICO name. Mother Dear thought the little green lizard was real, too — really alive, really talking (with a British accent, no less), and really intelligent.

Mom: How do they get him to do that? I've been watching him for years and he makes sense!

My brother and I came up with a good retort to that one:

Gecko: [Saying anything.]

Mom: How do they get him to do that?

My Brother and Me: I want to know why he speaks with a British accent!

Mom: [Furrows her brow and gets lost in thought.]

* * *

Commercials often take liberties with reality to make a point. One promoting a brand of chicken depicted a man stooped over and peering into an open refrigerator looking for something delicious to eat. His family discovered him immobilized in this position, frozen in time, and his wife quickly diagnoses his condition as a "refrigerator coma" and that the company's varieties of chicken are the cure.

Mom: I hope I never slip into a refrigerator coma.

Perception is reality. For Mother Dear, her reality was fluid, presented by the media and seen through dementia-colored glasses.

OBSESSIONS

When I heard a sentence that started with "I gotta do..." I knew there was an obsessive behavior on the horizon. "I gotta do the closets." "I gotta do the jewelry box." Translation: She was having an overwhelming desire to yank everything out of various storage spaces like she was on an archeological dig and scatter the contents across multiple rooms and pieces of furniture for inspection. She'd make a complete mess in the name of reorganization.

Once things were strewn about, she didn't have the first clue about how to put the items away. This was often met with incredulity that she'd actually caused the upset in the first place because she really didn't remember, or frustration that she knew it was her project but hadn't the faintest clue about how to finish. Ultimately the job of spending hours to tidy up fell to me.

The coat closet might be the target of the day. She would bring the contents in to me, sometimes one at a time, sometimes two or three items at a time, and show them to me.

Coats, shoes, boots, a dust buster, spare tiles from a mirrored wall. More often than not, the items made more than one trip in for my attention because she forgot what had been done. For example, she'd bring in a red coat, show it to me like she had discovered something on a fact-finding mission, and then bring it back to the closet. A blue jacket was the next find she'd show me. When she brought back the blue jacket, she rediscovered the red coat.

When this train would start down the tracks, I'd try to derail it at the beginning by redirecting her attention to something else. I'd talk about the pets or bring up any topic that would distract her and break the cycle. That was a futile effort. I imagined it to be like someone with Tourette's Syndrome trying to suppress a tick. They may be successful for a while but eventually the compulsive action makes its way to the surface regardless of how much concentration can be mustered.

Mom's process of rearranging repeated itself until she tired herself out. There was no reasoning with her so I just had to wait for her to get it out of her system.

One particular incident began with, "I gotta do that chest in the bedroom." The chest to which she referred was her large cedar chest that was filled with all sorts of linens and things. It was the hope chest from her marriage and I really wouldn't be surprised if the items contained within it were from then as well.

It had a latch on the front that she couldn't get open. The stars had aligned in my favor. The button on the front with a keyhole provided me with a convenient way out since I was able to shrug my shoulders and say I didn't know how to open it, either. It wasn't locked, it was just that she couldn't push the button in far enough to release the top, but that didn't stop me from telling her that she would need the key and it was anyone's guess where that was located. It was a plausible answer and one that she could understand. It frustrated her and it successfully delayed her ability to act on her compulsion.

One night, in the middle of the night, she must have figured out how to open it — by persistence and a bit of shear luck — because there was all manner of junk spread atop her bed and dresser in the morning.

The flotsam included a vintage mink stole. If you've never seen one of these, it's how popular mink stoles were made back in the "olden days," post World War II, when it was fashionable to wear mink wraps. The minks looked like they'd just been shot out back by Davy Crockett and sewed together by Betsy Ross. There were three minks attached neck to butt. The heads were still in place, skull-less with their eye sockets and mouths crudely sewn shut. I'm sure when my mother stepped out on the town with it draped around her shoulders, she felt like a million bucks and other ladies were envious.

The wrap was creepy but I was used to it since it had passed out of fashion and become a plaything around the house when I was growing up.

Several times after opening the chest, she brought the minks out to show me what she had found. "Now where would I wear something like this," she'd titter.

What had been a fetching accessory to a smart outfit in decades gone by became a fright in the middle of the night. All was well until she came in to get me. I must have been sleeping lightly because I awoke with the feeling that someone was in the room. She was standing over me and staring down at my face.

Mom: [Concerned.] There's something dead in my bed.

Me: [*Thinking* to myself.] Yeah, it's those God damn dusty minks you've been trotting around the house for the past week.

I got up and led her to the bedroom where I used the wall-mounted switch just inside the door to turn on the light.

Me: [Saying out loud to her.] Don't worry; it's just that mink stole you found in the cedar chest.

I placed the minks in a bureau drawer, returned to the den, and kept reminding myself that patience was a virtue as I drifted back to sleep.

After the cedar chest, Mom rediscovered her jewelry armoire and took everything out of it. There were rings, there were necklaces, and there were bracelets. There were earrings, there were stickpins, and there were brooches, too. Most of them were good as new. It was the collection she'd assembled from boutiques and stores, catalogs, and flea markets. Some were inherited, some were souvenirs, yet others had been a gift. All had a special moment where they'd been discovered and given her a lift.

Mom's jewelry bender had her finest gold strewn from one side of the living room to the other. Every piece was carefully inspected and she tried each of them on. It was like watching someone play dress up, or going shopping with someone who puts something on in the fitting room and then struts out to model it in a mini fashion show, seeking approval before buying. By the time Mom made it through the hundred items she'd found, she started in at the beginning because it all looked new again. The treasure trove of trinkets tempted her with the promise of shiny new revelations of gold, silver, and gems galore.

She insisted on showing me every piece. I would think to myself, "Yes, it's pretty, just like the last five times you showed it to me." If it weren't for the fact that it kept her occupied, I would have expressed a higher level of irritation.

After tiring of the project, she stood back and looked at the collection in total. She took a deep breath and sighed, basking in the brilliance of it all. She decided everything was so beautiful that it should be given away to someone who would appreciate each piece as much as she did. Jewelry should be worn, shown about, rather than cast into the darkness of a dresser.

It was an idea with which I didn't disagree. She had already given two pieces to a friend who sought and received my approval before accepting them. Then Mom threatened to put up a card table in the front yard to sell the rest. That would have been quite a spectacle.

I didn't put any of it back right away because the obsession needed to run its course. If I put it away too early, she would just drag it all back out again, so I saved myself the trouble and resulting aggravation. After three years of doing the caregiver gig, I had the hang of what and what not to do.

I was sitting on the couch with bracelets covering the center cushion.

Mom: [Pointing to the jewelry.] I'd like to know who got this all out.

Me: You did.

Mom: Oh sure, why am I always to blame?

I clearly needed to get better in tune with when she decided to play the blame game so I could get ahead of her in the conversation. It seemed like she was looking for an argument.

Me: Okaaaaaay, I did it.

Mom: Don't get smart with me.

When I realized what I'd said and how I said it, it was too late. If I had only said it was me that took the stuff out right from the start it would have thrown her off track. I'd spoken without really thinking, out of irritation, and I was too far in.

Whenever I would tell her she'd done something — and she didn't remember it because she didn't remember anything — she leaped right into defensive mode. She did it, you just couldn't convince her.

A subset of the "I gotta do..." was organizing anything that wasn't nailed down. Paperwork included. This was another activity that she managed to accomplish during the early hours of the morning — while she was up and I was asleep.

I had received an unsolicited mailing to subscribe to a pornographic magazine. Since moving home, I hadn't received any

X-rated material up until that point. It was one thing when I lived on my own, but porn can cause a bit of discomfort when living with the parental units. The company had likely obtained my contact information from a subscription mailing list rented from *The Advocate* magazine. For those unfamiliar with *The Advocate*, it's basically a gay version of Newsweek. Politics, news, entertainment, and lifestyle. It does not have naked pictures or erotica.

I opened the envelope and looked through the contents. I'm not above looking at free naked pictures even if I don't plan on buying them. Free naked photos are free naked photos, after all. When I finished giving them a thorough review, I placed the contents on top of a shredder where I disposed of sensitive materials such as pre-approved credit card offers.

Mom was already in bed so the "Sexual Materials Enclosed" envelope and its contents were saved for shredding at a later time. On the other side of the wall from the shredder is exactly where my Mom's head was when she was asleep. Out of courtesy, I didn't want to make any loud noise that might disturb her.

Now if I had been more prescient, I would have figured out where this was going to end. The papers weren't nailed down, and I was fully aware of what that could lead to, so it really was my own fault.

A day later I found the explicit photos of naked men among various papers and opened mail that Mother had collected and organized into nice neat stacks on the floor of the den. Knowing her process it dawned on me that she had looked at everything very closely to determine in which pile each piece should be placed.

Seeing a naked man must have been a shock. He was smiling into the camera, but still. Any flies on the wall would have had a great laugh over that. She never mentioned it. I immediately thought that it would be my luck that it would be the one thing she'd remember and blab it to persons unknown.

GARDENING FRUSTRATIONS

What is the dividing line between passion and obsession? The point where it transitions from healthy to unhealthy? What part could dementia play?

Mother Dear kept a meticulous yard, one of her enjoyable activities, when she was a stay-at-home Mom. Squaring up the hedges with the clippers, planting the annuals, and watering the grass. Standing bent at the waist, saving sore knees damaged from years of playing high school basketball, to weed flowerbeds for hours at a time. Wisps of hair framed her face while beads of perspiration rolled down her nose, dropping off the ball at the tip to the manicured lawn below.

She returned to a hands-on role in the yard when she retired. Retirement provided days summoning to be filled with activity, and that meant going outside and puttering around. She continued to relinquish the heavy work to the gardeners and went about doing the tedious detail work herself.

The problem with her yard work wasn't that she did it — she did a wonderful job and enjoyed it immensely — it was that her growing levels of dementia interfered with her brain's internal mechanism that told her to stop when she was overdoing it. The nature of her obsession kept her going from sunrise to sunset, rarely stopping to rest or rehydrate by drinking.

Couple Alzheimer's with an obsessive-compulsive penchant for picking at things at ground level and you've got a clean garden. There was always one more dandelion within sight that needed to be pulled. One more faded blossom to pinch. One more leaf to be picked up and so forth.

She was correct in her reasoning that it didn't take much effort; just a few seconds more to do it. It was this line of thinking that kept her going. It's like thinking you can eventually lift 500 pounds by starting low and adding one pound to the barbell each day. In the abstract, it seems reasonable that you should be able to lift a little more each day than you did the day before. In practice, there comes a day when you can't. And with gardening, there comes a time when one more weed is one too many.

Soldiering on until there wasn't any more to do relieved her from sitting in the house and thinking about any unfinished business. If she had stopped, her body might relax, but her mind would not. This compulsive behavior led to her physical collapse several times that we know of — probably more when no one was around. Heat and humidity have an easier victory over the body as years pass, exacting an incrementally larger toll on the human condition each year of age.

I was cleaning in the basement when the teenager from next door came running into the house yelling for me. "Your Mom fell down in the yard!" Neighbors across the street, nurses both, had come running to her aid when they witnessed her keel over. They were checking her vital signs and evaluating her status by the time I'd flown up the stairs, flung the screen door open to the furthest point of its hinges, and rushed to her side.

I ran back into the house and returned with an umbrella to shield her from the blazing sun and a glass of room temperature water. (Cold water can cause the stomach to cramp in people with heat exhaustion.) As I was helping her up, all she could think about was the twigs in her view that were just out of reach. She reached for them, trying to pick them up!

The dementia prevented her from remembering these dramas. Trying to use such a medical incident as part of a reasoned argument to get her to slow down meant nothing to her. It served as more fuel for the debate that would ensue where I banged my head against the brick walls in her mind. Her rebuttals being that she felt fine and I wasn't telling the truth. Dementia is a magician, making things disappear at will.

It was an ordinary Tuesday and Mother Dear took an afternoon break from her yard work and came into the house. She wandered into the den where I was working on the computer and she fell asleep on the couch behind me.

I slowly swiveled in the desk chair to check on her when I heard her rustling about. It wouldn't be unusual for her to be staring right back at me. She was in deep REM having the best dream of her life. She was picking up leaves in her sleep! Yes, she was literally moving her hands, picking and grabbing with her right hand and then transferring the imaginary leaves into her left hand where she collected them. In the yard, when she couldn't hold any more in her left hand, she'd make a little pile that I would dutifully pick up on a sweep of the yard in the evening.

Mom had spent the day doing yard work, part of a weeklong marathon. I tried to discourage the amount of time she spent by hiding all her tools — the pruning clippers and rakes were placed out of sight on a high shelf. I kept checking in, telling her to come in the house to get out of the sun because she was over exerting again. I tempted her with cool lemonade and pleaded for her to sit in a lawn chair to enjoy the fruits of her labor. Her response was, "Who says I'm not enjoying it?" It was, I conceded, an excellent point.

The next day, however, she would pay the price. She was completely spaced out and had pain in her fingers and neck. She didn't know where she was, what a "yard" was, or much of anything else. The physical activity drained her mental activity.

Therein lied my dilemma. Should I let her work in the yard, which clearly brought her happiness, exercise, focus, and contentment knowing that the end result could be a disaster? Or should I up her meds and seat her like a zombie in front of the television? I chose to avoid the fights, let her do what she liked best, and enjoy the remaining years of her life. My father dropped dead in our backyard doing the same thing and everyone said, "At least he died doing what he loved."

I found enjoyment in the same things, grounding myself in the earth and taking pride as bulbs planted in October burst forth as spring flowers. I staged the plantings so there was always a beautiful star in the garden regardless of season, beaming with pride at each clump of posies that were a replacement for raising the children I never had. I saved my best efforts for when the weather was glorious — warm and low humidity.

As I worked my way around the yard planting flowers, Mother Dear followed a couple days later and pulled them all up. She confused the small sprouts as "weeds." Weeds were everything that looked dead, new sprouts, or any plant that looked out of place.

I had planted seven bare-root rose bushes; five climbers along the neighbor's chain link fence that separated our yards and two hybrid teas among the daffodils on the north side of the house. One of them was my favorite Double Delight, with pretty pink and white rose blossoms that were wonderfully fragrant, smelling exactly how you would imagine a rose to smell.

Two of the climbers didn't make it to summer as Mom pulled them up before they could get established because they "were dead." The remaining plants did eventually bud and grow but the harsh cold of winter wasn't kind to them. The following spring, Mom gazed at them from the window, fixated. She couldn't wait to yank them up. The day came when she got to them when I wasn't around. I found them on the lawn, dirt clinging to their roots. Her task was complete.

These were the things that frustrated me. It made me angry that things had progressed to the point where I worked hard to make the yard beautiful and she followed behind me and ruined it. More than once I had the feeling, "Why do I even try?"

The dog days of summer brought in one storm front after another, the heavy black clouds approaching from the west. All afternoon and evening, the Emergency Broadcast System was hard at work sending out warning tones on the television. At dusk, a woman with a robotic tin voice alerted us that storms producing quarter size hail were forming and to take cover. She also informed me of something that I didn't know — lightning strikes can occur 15 miles from the center of the storm. If you can hear thunder that means there's a danger of being struck!

There was a loud clap of thunder that sent Chiquita running through the house, ears folded back and flat against her head. She eventually settled in the bathroom to hide. I began taking an inventory and remembered that Pooh Pooh had gone outside after the storm that passed through earlier that afternoon. I hadn't seen Mother Dear in a while, either. I rushed through the house calling for her, going from room to room, and looking on the floor to see if she had fainted or collapsed since she wasn't answering.

She wasn't in the house. I found her picking up leaves off the front lawn, in the dark, with flashes of lightning strikes and the crashing sounds of thunder all around. The storm was severe, making me afraid to go out in the yard to get her. There she stood with the damn leaves clenched in her left fist. I yelled at her to get in the house. She'd take five steps, then stop and pick up a few more leaves. A feeling of relief settled over me when she finally made her way inside.

I had to remind myself that she just couldn't help it.

For as long as I could remember, this was a woman that used to take to her bed, pull the covers over her head, and cry during any thunderstorm. When she was a child, there had been a lightning strike close to the house that sent electric current through her home. My Grandma was knocked out of her chair, her feet having been on a metal strip that held kitchen floor linoleum in place. Mom had been afraid ever since. The dementia had made her forget her extreme fear of lightning storms.

Chasing Mom around the yard made it clearer that I needed help in managing her.

HIRING AN AIDE

My mood began to parallel that of my mother, slowly rolling down an alley of despair with seemingly no end. There was still a speck of light at the end, the sun going down over the horizon. Its brightness, once extinguished, would hail the end of the manageability of my festering emotions.

Days passed and I wouldn't feel like eating until dinnertime. My weight loss cried out for nourishment but my mind couldn't motivate my body to consume anything. My periods of sleep stretched on for 16 hours a day yet I never seemed to catch up because I had to sleep lightly and didn't get proper rest. There wasn't a drop of energy left in the bucket. As they say, "My get up and go, just got up and went."

The only effort my body seemed complicit in making was a dedication to keeping my gut tied in a twist — a double helix of agita. The knots weren't the butterflies that flutter inside in anticipation of a phone call from a new love. These were spasms that kept my core locked tight. The tautness in my stomach prevented anything from entering from above. The lack of food also deprived me of energy.

The spiral of no sleep, no food, and no energy wound tighter and tighter as it reached the point where the pent up tension was going to unleash like a coiled spring released from a comedian's can of nuts.

One of the most significant words you will hear in the counseling of caregivers is "respite." Professionals emphasize how important it is to take breaks and get some rest. Humans push themselves to take on too much; particularly those with martyr and Type A personalities, thinking their shoulders are broad enough to carry the weight of the world. Even the Energizer pink bunny that races across the screen thumping his bass drum eventually needs to pull in for a pit stop, recharging its internal power source to keep going.

A change in surroundings is strongly encouraged, whether it's a simple trip to the library for some quiet reading, a walk down the street to clear the mind, having coffee at a local café for some casual social interaction, or a more sustained absence like a vacation. Time away can seem selfish in the mindset of many caregivers but there's no sense in them going down with the ship. The more energy one has, the more one can continue to give. The investment in respite reaps future benefits for everyone.

Many caregivers are prevented from following this simple advice because they are presented with the problem of finding a resource to take care of the patient during the interim. A lack of support could be the reason for feeling trapped in the first place. A catch-22.

If family and friends aren't available, checking for resources can yield many ways to get assistance. The community's social safety net, such as church congregations and organizations such as Meals on Wheels, can be tapped for support. The government's safety net also offers assistance. Any research should start with the local County Department of the Aging or similar agency. They may even have a program to pay for the patient to be placed in an assisted living facility on a short-term basis to lift the financial burden. Or, there may be an option for daycare that eases the burden of a continuous time commitment.

I began touring local assisted living centers and nursing homes. (This is a topic that I discuss in further detail in an upcoming chapter.) The high costs were surprising.

My mother wasn't eligible for a monthly stipend from the Veterans Benefits Administration. It would have been available from my father's service during World War II. However, her liquid assets and income, which included Social Security and mandatory disbursements from retirement accounts, were too high. The VA benefit was a reasonable sum and could contribute a large chunk to the cost of care for many of our veterans and their families. Unfortunately, she didn't qualify.

Mother Dear had been smart with her money. There was plenty for her needs as a result of investments made with the advice of a keen financial planner. A small contribution to a diverse portfolio of stocks, bonds, and annuities had grown exponentially during the go-go run up of the stock market during the 90's. At retirement time, everything had been moved to low risk financial instruments and she avoided the losses suffered by so many during the subsequent financial instabilities. We were lucky that she was able to cover her own expenses.

After watching her father waste away in a nursing home from Alzheimer's disease, while her mother struggled with the finances to support his care, my mother purchased a Long Term Care (LTC) insurance policy. In New York State, and perhaps elsewhere, the government had joined forces with insurance companies to provide LTC policies to defray their Medicaid expenses.

Here's how my mother's policy was structured. All insurance companies, state laws, and policies are different. The following is for reference only; each individual contract should be reviewed accordingly:

- The insured person paid yearly premiums from the time it was bought until the time a claim was approved.

- There was a formula embedded into the contract that increased the benefits with the cost of living. This helped avoid policies that wouldn't pay enough for care when they were used many years later. For example, say a policy purchased in 1990 paid $50 per day. When a claim was made in 2010, twenty years later, the cost of care equivalent to 1990 might be $100 per day. The yearly increase in benefits ensured that the payout was closer to the future cost of care. Without this, the insured might still have to liquidate assets, the avoidance of which is one of the main reasons to buy the policy.

- Premiums were set by the insurance company's actuaries. The younger the insured was at the time the policy was bought, the lower the premiums were to incentivize people to buy into the system earlier. The insurance company compensated for the lower premium by collecting payments over a longer timeframe.

How did the insurance company win? They're betting that the insured dies before making a claim on the policy or dies before the full benefit of the policy has been paid. It's like car insurance in reverse, where they risk that the insured won't have an accident that requires a payout larger than the total of the premiums paid. The driver wagers that they will have a need for the policy by having an accident.

How did the state win? They mitigated their outlays by sharing the cost of elder care with the insurance company. The state didn't pay for the initial costs. As with the insurance company, if the insured passed away before the policy had paid out its maximum benefit, the state's Medicaid plan hadn't paid anything.

How did the purchaser/insured win? Their assets were protected should long-term care be required. If the maximum payout specified in the contract was reached, Medicaid began coverage at the same rate of payment that the policy was paying rather than their standard minimum. Liquidation of assets is not required.

My mother purchased this policy to improve the level of care in future years and reduce the potential burden on her family — not to protect her assets although that was a compelling side benefit.

Without this type of policy, assets must be liquidated and spent before government assistance begins. In other words, if someone ends up in a nursing home, the government doesn't pay anything toward his or her care until they are unable to pay for the care themselves — having sold their house, emptied bank accounts, and essentially spent their children's inheritance.

After the elderly person is broke, the government only reimburses a set amount per day for their care. This is only enough to cover the charges for the most basic facilities. If the patient's family had money, were generous, and they weren't estranged from the parents somewhere along the way, they might make up whatever gap existed between the level of care afforded by the Medicaid payments for a higher level of living and care. Based on what I've witnessed, I recommend planning ahead and not counting on the future kindness of others — including family.

When it came time to get assistance, I read the LTC policy and met with an agency representative. It paid a maximum benefit of $120 per day for in-home care or an assisted living facility. The payout jumped to $250 per day for a nursing home. There was a deductible time period of 30 individual days of care received, regardless of the amount of time billed each day. Two hours of help a day counted as much as eight hours of help towards the deductible time period. Since this was out of pocket, we went with the minimum of two hours and increased it when the deductible had been met.

At the time, Mom's condition and requirements were getting beyond my sole (and soul) capabilities. She needed help and I desperately needed relief from the crushing daily grind. My brother and I decided to go incrementally on her care, starting slowly with an in-home aide and increasing those hours as time went by. As Mother

Dear's condition deteriorated, we would consider placing her where a more in-depth level of care could be provided. The idea was to keep her in familiar surroundings as long as it was feasible and I was capable.

To activate the reimbursement of payments from her LTC policy, the insurance company required that an assessment be performed to verify the legitimacy of the claim. During the initial evaluation, I answered all of the questions because Mom wasn't capable. She did make some colorful contributions under her breath with comments such as "He's full of shit" or "That never happened," after each of my replies.

I filled out a myriad of paperwork and her primary care physician was required to complete a special form. After that, the claim was approved and we were assigned to an account manager. Our representative was first-rate and knowledgeable as she guided me through the process quickly, pleasantly, and got everything set up without any problems. It couldn't have gone any smoother.

I was given the names of three home care agencies in our area, one of which they had negotiated a discount on the price. A quick search on the Internet didn't turn up any other recommendations so I settled on those three as my starting point. A neighbor that had gone through the same thing didn't present a positive picture when she said, "they're all the same" and "they're all flakes."

I built a spreadsheet, as I do for just about everything, and started conducting my phone interviews. Filling in the grid with the questions and answers would organize the information in a way that would facilitate relevant comparisons. I asked about rates, availability, qualifications, etc. At the end of each call, I requested that the company send literature and a rate card.

There were several tiers of assistance available: companions who kept company, personal assistants who tended to errands, and home health care aides with varied medical training. Each person and agency was a bit different in what they were willing to do or offer. These are low paying positions after the agency takes their cut.

Meticulously defining specific needs and requirements up front ensures that everyone's expectations are met. Select a provider that can meet long-term requirements because these services may be needed for an extended period of time.

A list of "must do" items should be made before starting the interviews. Here's a list of items to consider:

- Will this person need to administer pills? Injections? Other special medical requirements? A companion is not qualified to do this.

- Will this person need to prepare meals? How many? Are there special dietary needs? Should you consider a program like Meals on Wheels?

- Will this person need to do any housework? Most will do light cleaning like dishes and tidying up. If you need a maid, hire a maid.

- Will this person need to provide transportation to hair or doctor appointments?

- Will this person need to be bi-lingual?

- Will this person need to assist with dressing, showering, and/or toileting? An investment in special equipment like a shower chair, shower wand, and handrails may be required.

- Are there pets in the house? Are they friendly? Who is responsible for their care? Quite a few people have allergies so animals can be problematic.

- Are there any smokers in the house? Many people refuse to work in a smoking environment.

There were some roadblocks I hadn't anticipated. I discovered that one agency didn't have any contacts "in our area." We were in a suburb and I hadn't considered that transportation could be a factor. There's no bus line, which presented a problem for aides that couldn't afford a car.

It seemed that all of the agencies essentially pulled talent from the same pool of caregivers, so I chose the one with the discounted rate. It really boiled down to the individual that showed up at the door and the price paid didn't seem to correlate with that. The good ones were paid the same rate as the bad ones. Price didn't guarantee quality.

Here in upstate New York, the going agency rate was around $20 per hour. Weekends were 50¢ more per hour, with holidays and overtime at 1.5 times the corresponding rate with a maximum of $100 per day.

We contracted for a home health care aide because of Mom's

fainting spells and seizure-like episodes. We wanted a qualified person with her in case anything happened when I ventured away from the house.

After opening the claim, we fulfilled the 30 days of care deductible at two hours a day then increased the hours to five a day once the insurance coverage began.

Aide #1

A light blue Buick family sedan pulled into the driveway. Rust from salty winter roads had corroded the chrome that outlined the wheel wells. The engine coughed with a hesitation after she turned off the key, straining to keep running despite the lack of an electrical charge.

Christy was young, in her early 20's, heavy set, with her hair pulled tightly into a pony tail that fell onto the collar of a plain white polyester frock. Black polyester pants and white shoes with thick rubber soles completed her standard-issue ensemble.

She was a bit unsure of herself, speaking softly and averting her dark brown eyes to avoid any contact with mine.

It was a slow ramp up. Mom had difficulty getting used to a stranger coming into the house. She wasn't afraid of this unknown presence, just confused. I answered Mom's questions of "Who's that woman who comes here?" and "Why is she coming here?" hundreds of times. The repetition afforded me the chance to reinforce Christy's name, hoping that it would lodge somewhere in the topsy-turvy labyrinth of Mom's memory cells. I reasoned that if she knew her name, she wouldn't feel so unfamiliar.

In the grand scheme of all possible jobs, our situation was an easy gig. There was no arithmetic or physical labor involved. Put in your five hours by showing up in the early afternoon, watch some television, serve Mom a bowl of ice cream, wash some dishes in the sink, and dial 9-1-1 if there was an emergency. If she were able to convince Mother Dear to take a shower, and then assist her, I would have considered it a huge bonus. For the most part, I was available as a backup and problem solver, working on freelance design projects on the computer in the den. I kept the door closed to provide some sense of separation and privacy but I was always there if needed.

Christy came three days a week for two months and then vanished. Our caseworker at the agency reported that she had quit, never having called to let them know. We weren't her only clients; others in more dependent situations were left without coverage. Months later, I saw her perusing fruits and vegetables in the produce department of the supermarket. I steered my cart clear, leaving her alone to evaluate the carefully arranged selection of polished red, yellow, and green apples on display.

While very nice, I felt she was a bit too young and introverted, and had difficulty relating to my mother. Her disappearance was a blessing in disguise as it opened the position for Marilyn.

Aide #2

The replacement aide was a friend of our family that Mom had known for decades. The niece of a neighbor, Marilyn was in her early 60's and belonged to the Ladies Auxiliary of the local volunteer fire department at the same time that Mom had years ago. They had common interests and her age was closer to my mother's.

Even though she was older, Marilyn's appearance seemed younger than Christy's. Her tops always had some splash of color, usually mixed with floral or geometric designs. Her glasses were small, round, and in-style while her brown hair was cut short, tousled, and easily maintained.

There wasn't a timid bone in her body, her bundle of high-energy personality practically making its way into a room before her physicality. Boisterous and up-to-speed with current events, she could comfortably engage in just about any conversation.

She was a chatterbox and that kept Mother Dear entertained. She talked to Mom, recounting old times they shared at dances and banquets, and discussed all of the friends and acquaintances who had crossed their paths along the way. Mom could still remember flashes of these fleeting times. They were like vague snippets clipped from the magazine of her life. These discussions drew upon things that her long-term memory could still access. Her short-term memory was completely non-existent by then, having succumbed to the ravages of the disease.

Besides the years of experience that she brought to the job, Marilyn possessed the ability to relate having taken care of her own elderly parents. She was a parent of three herself, two boys and a girl, and relished in that role as well as that of grandmother. Being a caregiver was in her nature.

We all got along famously. Mom liked her, and most importantly, she trusted her. She was able to convince Mom that Wednesdays were shower days. Marilyn had an easier time of it. First, she was experienced. Second, she was a non-related female and she helped

Mom in the shower more than I felt comfortable doing. Third, we brought the shower chair back and re-installed the hand-held shower wand at Marilyn's request and they worked wonderfully. As long as Mom wasn't responsible for using them, they were the perfect remedy to many of her fears. The process flowed better, and shortened the event, which reduced the stress on Mom.

A trick Marilyn used was to tell Mom they were going to "wash her hair." Even though they showered, it worked because Mom associated fear with the word "shower" but was fine with the alternate semantics.

Marilyn's arrival was pure luck of the draw that I attributed to the good karma I had built up since moving back to assume the caregiver role. Mother Dear and I weren't the only people delighted with her — her agency named her "Employee of the Year," an award that was much deserved. She proved compassionate, friendly, and dependable.

WTEN, the local ABC television affiliate, came to our house to film a piece on Marilyn for the evening news. The story was about the effect of high gas prices on folks who drove to their various job assignments throughout the day. They asked me to do an on-camera interview but I declined because the story wasn't about us. It appeared at the top of the 6 o'clock newscast and provided some excitement for the day!

* * *

I overheard Mother talking about my brother and me to Marilyn.

Mom: I love those two guys. They're great guys.

That made me feel good.

I LOVE A PARADE

The conviction with which something is told can easily blur the lines between what's right and wrong, what's real and imagined, what's true and false. It's the mark of a con man, liar, or dementia sufferer. If the speaker displays complete confidence in their tale it's likely that the listener will believe it. Such candor can overcome a listener's instinct to pause and perform a quick double check with their common sense, which is the psyche's primary level of determining the authenticity of a story.

Part of the service provided by the home aide assistance firm was a no-cost monthly visit by a nurse. This was a really nice convenience that reduced our need for office visits to the doctor. A professional checked simple things like blood pressure, heart rate, and temperature. The aide also monitored any changes in condition during her visits and reported the condition of the patient to the agency for follow-up by the nurse if need be.

From their standpoint, it was good business practice that they received a general assessment of physical health and served as a great safety check for clients that only had minimal assistance. While my mother had the ideal situation of someone living with her full time, most didn't. Some couldn't afford better care, insurance only covered minimal help, and/or they were left alone by their children to fend for themselves.

Others could be in an abusive situation that required intervention by authorities. There are people who are just plain rotten and take out their frustrations with the world on the defenseless people around them. The strains placed on someone who is a caregiver to a person that requires advanced levels of attention could trigger folks to behave in an abusive manner as stress builds. Agencies are on-site and can provide those patients with a lifeline, an added level of security for those most vulnerable.

Nurse: [To mom.] So how have you been?

Mom: Oh, pretty good.

Nurse: What have you been up to?

Mom: Well, I was in a parade the other day on the road just up over the hill.

Mom pointed behind the house in the direction of the main road where town parades were usually held. As a member of the Ladies Auxiliary, Mom had participated in many parades.

Each year, surrounding fire departments were invited to participate for awards and trophies based on how they appeared in the parade. Attention was paid to dress uniforms, uniformity of marching, and condition of their apparatus. Spiraling lights on top of the fire engines' cabs were always on and the periodic yelp of the sirens brought smiles to the families that lined the route. Most trucks were fire engine red except for the occasional one painted chartreuse.

Those that weren't selected by the judges for fit and finish during the parade were able to make it up during an afternoon of competitions designed to gauge their fire fighting skills. Climbing a façade to douse an oil fire in a barrel, an obstacle course, unrolling/rolling hoses, ending with a tug-o-war provided some exciting activities. A stopwatch rather than the eye of judges determined the winners of the trophies.

The festivities ended in a carnival in the evening where esprit de corps was celebrated around games of chance, B-B-Q chicken dinners, and the beer garden.

Nurse: Wow! That's great!

The nurse looked at me with a smile and nodded her affirmation of what a wonderful thing she'd just heard about Mom's recent escapades. I shook my head 'no' and winked behind my mother's back.

Nurse: [Blushing.] Oh.

Sometimes things are too good to be true. Mom believed she was in a parade and said so convincingly. I wondered if her stories were like dreams, only that they occurred during the day while awake.

* * *

The fair people of the great Northeast can count on at least one terrible ice storm a year. They usually occur in late March or early April on the cusp of winter's transition to spring. It's a way that I've always gauged whether the cold months are truly behind us. It signals that winter will be left behind after its last hurrah and the crocuses will begin to sprout and peak up from the soil to welcome spring. Sometimes the daffodils pushed their way up through the last vestiges of snow.

In those storms, the limber trees swooned to the ground as they succumbed to the added weight of a half-inch of freezing rain coating every exposed surface. Limbs and branches broke off of those that weren't as flexible, filling the eerie silence with the sounds of snapping and the crashing made as the boughs fell to earth and took down anything in their path. Sometimes utility wires.

An unusual December storm hit the area and caused an 18-hour power outage, lasting nearly a full day from 3 a.m. until 9 p.m., before the power company's line crews were able to clean up the debris and repair the resulting damage. There were an estimated 217,000 of our closest friends and neighbors in the same predicament.

Power, phone, and cable television lines were brought down from their poles throughout the area. It was a modern 21st century blackout with our 3-in-1 television/phone/Internet services out of commission. I found some D-size batteries and turned on an old radio for news reports and some entertainment. Voices and tunes hissed and crackled from the dusty old speaker, not having received any transmissions in years.

The oil-based furnace in the basement required electricity to ignite the burner and activate the forced air fan so we were without heat. The last time a storm of that magnitude hit was two decades earlier and my brother had bought a gas-powered generator for the house to be prepared. Being in the attached garage, it's quite convenient, and stays plugged directly into the house wiring via a special outlet so everything works the same as if the power were coming from the outside lines when the generator is running.

The foresight of having this in place allowed us to run the furnace as the temperature outside was down to 5°F. The generator ran for about an hour on a full tank of gas, which was enough time to get the house warmed up. Things would cool off after about three hours, requiring me to refill the tank and start it up again. Items that drew a big surge of power, such as heating elements in the electric oven, toaster, and hair dryer, were not used.

In the meantime, I sat quietly in the candlelight. I laid down on the sofa and fell asleep at about 8 p.m. Mother came into the den shortly thereafter and practically sat on my feet at the end of the couch in the dark. She was awake and looking for company.

I tried to reposition myself and keep on sleeping but Mom had no intentions of moving. Being alone in the dark had her disoriented and lonely. I asked where she wanted to go, and she said she wanted to be near me. My mother's bed is a California King size where she and my Dad used to sleep. I ended up sleeping on his side and she on hers. It was a great solution because each of us got what we needed. She got company. I got sleep.

It worked out well although she kept waking me up by talking in her sleep. The apple doesn't fall far from the tree, as far as that goes, because I'm famous for speaking my portion of my dreams aloud. Her best line:

Mom: We gotta get these cattle out of the road!

Dream analysis would be an interesting line of work.

* * *

The people who live in our area have learned to prepare for these disruptions in electrical service by stocking up on candles. They aren't just used as decoration or to provide homes with various scents of nature or of the season. Here, they're functional, too, providing light during an electrical outage.

We kept a bowl full of tea light candles at the end of the kitchen counter, conveniently located in the event of a short power outage. The generator was only used when absolutely necessary. Several candles would be lit for each room, flickering away the hours and casting shadows on the darkened walls, before the lights came back on.

The bowl of candles had been placed next to a bowl of cellophane-wrapped hard cinnamon candies. One day I was shocked when I discovered the bowl of candles had been moved from the counter to the couch with a Yankee Candle Potpourri Tart candle on the cushion next to it. The cellophane had been removed and teeth marks were evident in the wax on the side where a nibble had been taken. The candles were shaped like a little tart that you'd find in the display case of the grocery's bakery section or the pages of a Martha Stewart cook book. I can't imagine that it was too appetizing since it was green and smelled like eucalyptus — perhaps if it were strawberry scented Mom would have eaten the whole thing. Dementia is a bully, pushing common sense right out the window!

* * *

Mom came to the point where it was impossible for her to prepare anything to eat. There had been an intermediate phase where she could heat items in the toaster oven or frozen dinners in the microwave oven.

Mother Dear emerged from the kitchen with a frozen Lean Cuisine in her hands. I watched her fidget with it and wondered where this was all going. She opened the box, removed the tray, and peeled the cellophane from the top.

Me: What are you doing?

Mom: I want some ice cream.

Me: That's a chicken and rice dinner.

Mom: [Stern and irritated.] I don't know what I'm doing.

Me: Well let's get you some ice cream.

We went back out to the kitchen and I opened the freezer. I pointed to the half-gallon container of her favorite Pecan Praline.

Me: Here's where the ice cream is.

I pulled it out and set it on the counter to spoon up a dish for her.

Mom: Don't you have anything smaller? I like those little cups.

Mom held up her thumb and index finger to signal about four inches.

Me: Oh, you want pudding?

I opened the refrigerator and pointed to a pudding cup.

Mom: Yes. [Smiling]

All her meals were now ready-to-eat. Pre-packaged salads and meals were her sustenance. She would "make" pudding by peeling off the foil cover. She could unwrap candy placed on the counter, such as Hershey's Kisses, and eat them. As time went on, she wasn't able to find her favorite ice cream in the freezer because she didn't understand the concept of it being located on top of the refrigerator.

* * *

I heard the water running in the kitchen sink and the clanking together of plates and glasses. Mom was doing the dishes. After five minutes, I went out to check on her progress.

The left basin was full of soapy water with about half of the remaining dishes submerged. The right basin had the rest drying in an upright plastic rack. The dishes were wet but still dirty.

She had placed the dirty ones in the soapy water, then rinsed them, and placed them in the rack to dry. She had forgotten the washing step.

Me: How are you making out?

I figured I would just re-wash everything the next morning while she was still in bed.

Mom: [Beginning to cry.] Something's wrong. The dishes are still dirty and I don't know why.

She was frustrated. She knew she was doing something wrong but her brain just skipped the washing portion and kept her from seeing it even when examining the process for the problem.

* * *

My Grandmother ended up in a nursing home after suffering a stroke. She had been in her favorite chair working on a crossword puzzle to exercise her mind. The stroke was so severe that she lost all feeling in the left side of her body.

One day she was struggling in her hospital bed, reaching across her stomach with her right hand and pushing her numb left arm off the side of the bed. The right side of her brain was telling her that there was someone dead (the left side of her body) next to her and she was trying to get the dead body out of her bed. Her mind refused to understand any explanation regarding the stroke and that the "dead body" was her other half. Because the stroke was so severe, as far as the right side of her brain was concerned, the left side didn't exist and was not a part of her body.

The brain is so complex and works in mysterious ways!

PHYSICAL HEALTH

With dementia patients, the focus is often on their mental health yet their aging bodies are just as susceptible to the physical ailments associated with getting old. It is hard to determine exactly what's wrong when they're sick because they can't clearly communicate the problem. Mom also used inventive ways to get attention by accentuating things. Cases in point:

- She could make her teeth chatter and body shiver when she said she was cold. And it was 85°F and everyone else was sweating.
- She said she couldn't talk and acted like she had a thick swollen tongue.
- She grabbed the doorjamb and said "I'm gonna go down" from being dizzy.
- She talked like she had a stuffy nose when she needed a tissue, even though her nose was running.

I never knew when she was really sick or when she wasn't sick. Her dementia said she was and perhaps she was doing it for attention, or some other reason. The common conundrum of perception vs. reality. It added a layer of stress on me since I had the responsibility of trying to figure out which it was, and if I ignored something that turned out to be real, the blame would rest on my shoulders.

* * *

A hidden cause of Alzheimer's-like symptoms could be a malfunctioning thyroid gland. To eliminate an overactive thyroid as a possibility for Mom's maladies, they administered a radioactive iodine pill. The radiation collected in the thyroid and effectively "killed" the gland. To the delight of Big Pharma, the patient is then on thyroid replacement medication for the rest of their life. In my Mom's case, the prescription was Synthroid.

Every six months we had to go to the endocrinologist to make sure her hormone levels were as they should be. After the doctor listened to her heart through his stethoscope, manually felt the thyroid gland in her throat, and checked her blood pressure, it was off to have some blood drawn in a different part of the office. I made a joke about the guy poking her with the needle. Mom raised her hand on the arm without the tourniquet, lifted her middle finger, and said, "That's for you."

If her blood pressure was a tad high, there was no cause for alarm because she suffered from fainting spells that had been diagnosed as a drop in blood pressure when she stood up. She was on a prescription to keep this from happening but she refused to keep her compression stockings on to force the blood up to the brain instead of settling in her legs. Having blood pressure on the higher side could be a good thing.

These appointments always went smoothly with the office running like clockwork. Mother Dear really liked her physician who was a very personable guy from Russia with a trimmed beard and easy smile. Low key, pleasant…I liked him, too.

* * *

Mother Dear had a sore tooth that had been giving her intermittent trouble for some time because of a cavity that extended below the gum line near the jawbone. Based on the dentist's advice and the overall health of the tooth, he said it would eventually need to come out but we decided to let it go until it became too sore to tolerate. That time came.

We made an appointment with an oral surgeon to have it removed because she had unusual bone growth (mandibular tori) along the inside of her bottom jaw. A root canal or anything else to save the tooth would be too painful for what it would gain.

Until we met with the surgeon, she was placed on an antibiotic to reduce the inflammation and get the infection under control. She also had a prescription for the pain and I bought some Orajel to numb the area when the pain was at its worst.

There were times when the pain was so acute that she would curl up into a fetal position, hold her jaw, and cry. She complained that it felt like there was a knife in her mouth and the pain would shoot back to her ear.

Touching it made her wince and whimper. So what would she do? Constantly touch it! When I told her that she was only causing it to hurt by poking at it, I received the familiar, "Sure, it's always my fault" refrain.

As the pain increased, I called our neighbor Judy who is a dental hygienist to make an assessment as another opinion. Given the symptoms, she said it could be any number of things, including an ear infection or Temporomandibular Joint Disorder (TMJ). She agreed that we had been taking the correct course of action.

Mom called me into the bedroom the following morning because she had awoken in pain. I retrieved the antibiotic, two pain pills, and a glass of water from the kitchen. She was in agony and needed assistance sitting up, drinking, and swallowing the medication. She was confused, not sure how to drink from the glass, and wondering if she was at home.

I managed to get her upright and seated on the side of the bed. My brother had dropped in and came in to help. To distract her, he mentioned Simba the stuffed lion that sat on a chair next to her bed.

Mom: [Scowling at the lion.] Stop looking at me.

My brother talked about how nice the lion was to her and that he was just like the other two (live) cats in the house. That changed her tune.

Mom: [Smiling at the lion.] He's so cute. I just love him!

The pain medication took affect and she reported that she felt much better.

The appointment for the tooth extraction came and went with minimal disruption. The worst part was that the temperature outside was 12°F and windy. My brother acted as our chauffeur so we were able to get out of the car directly in front of the building to minimize the amount of walking on ice and exposure to the frigid cold.

We arrived at the office on time and she was in the dental chair within 10 minutes. My brother and I were instructed to wait in the reception area and the whole procedure was completed in five minutes.

I had prepared myself for a big scene but it went so smoothly that she didn't think they'd done anything!

Then, after we arrived at home, she said they had removed the wrong tooth because it was still bothering her. Uh oh. That was not the time to spring that little tidbit on us. The surgeon had, indeed, pulled the tooth with the decay that was suspected of causing all of the problems, Mom just didn't realize it because there was still some discomfort.

The spells where she would rock with her knees clutched to her chest because of the pain were over. She poked at it with her tongue a bit, which was to be expected, and that was the end. Or so we thought.

A week later, she started sporadically complaining of distress. I hypothesized that there was a fragment from the extracted tooth caught below the gum and it was working its way out. I wasn't too worried. My brother had a chip from a tooth find its way to the surface 30 years after he'd had his wisdom teeth removed!

As the days went by, her complaints of pain returned and became more frequent and more severe. With dementia patients, it's often the caregiver's job to gauge the level at which they are really feeling pain. Is the pain located where they say it is? What is the actual severity since everything is a 10 on a scale of 1-10 when you ask? It could be all or partly attributed to a figment of their dementia. How can a tooth continue to hurt when it had already been removed?

It had now been two weeks since her surgery and she was up all night holding her jaw. By the morning, the day before Christmas, she was doubled over and crying so I called her regular dentist for advice. It figured that this couldn't happen during normal business hours, rather on an emergency holiday basis. Medical emergencies don't care about the calendar when they occur. The first visit regarding the tooth had been a month before. That was the day after Thanksgiving, so at least Mother Dear was consistent in her holiday discontent.

She sat at the kitchen table and listened as I tracked down the doctor on the phone and made the appointment. No longer was her hand along her jaw — the pain miraculously had gone away. She started jabbering about the cats and looked at me with confusion when I ask her about her sudden lack of pain. "What pain?" She'd been on death's door bed minutes before, but when I found her some medical attention, she had no idea what I was talking about. I just wanted to scream!

Regardless, to the dentist we went. The dentist said that the area where the tooth had been extracted looked pink and that was a good indication of healing. The culprit was probably food or something caught down in the hole where the tooth's roots had been. He placed a probe down inside and it wasn't healed over so that seemed to be a reasonable diagnosis. There was a bit of blood on the probe further indicating that it wasn't healing like it should.

He instructed her to frequently rinse with warm salt water and he put her on the antibiotic Keflex. I requested something more powerful for the pain since the Naproxen wasn't helping during the worst flare-ups. He prescribed Tylenol-3 and I hoped that would help her sleep at night, too. I had successfully modified her routine so that she was sleeping at night and awake during the day but these marathon trips to painville during the early morning hours had negated all that effort. Her internal body clock was back out of whack.

The trouble continued despite the after-care and new medication so we went back to the oral surgeon. After recounting everything that had happened since our last visit, he inspected the extraction area and said it had healed fine. If she was continuing to have pain, it wasn't due to the tooth, which meant it was likely related to the nerve.

Next up was an appointment to see a neurologist. Months had passed and we were still dealing with the original problem — except she had one tooth fewer than when we started.

The neurologist correctly diagnosed the problem as Trigeminal Neuralgia which is described as sharp electric-like spasms, lasting a few seconds or longer. It is caused by the inflammation of the trigeminal nerve that delivers feeling to the face and surface of the eye. The condition usually affects older adults and no direct cause can be found.

The remedy was a prescription for an anti-seizure medication that had a secondary application for trigeminal neuralgia.

The months-long odyssey of pain was coupled with this lengthy investigation of the problem. Trial and error would have taken place on a regular person. However, dementia patients can't reliably convey what's really going on. The process is murkier. Thankfully we'd found the solution and brought her much needed relief. It all seemed obvious when the ordeal had finally come to an end. Hindsight is always 20/20.

* * *

Mom was experiencing quite a bit of pain in the mornings. She would come out of the bedroom holding her stomach and saying she "needed to go to the hospital," "wanted to die," or other ways to describe how much discomfort she was in with an upset stomach and nausea. She didn't want to eat and was sleeping a lot. I took her temperature and it was 97°F. A little low, but still okay. There was a virus going around and my brother and I thought it could be that.

A couple days went by and she refused to eat anything and drinking was infrequent as well. She was less disoriented by the middle of the week and able to eat half of an egg salad sandwich and drink some ginger ale. That worked a couple of days in a row and I coaxed her with some French fries. She was weak but improving. I was giving her Tums for the upset stomach. I considered that she was fighting acid indigestion based on the stomach pain and all the burping.

After another weekend of no food and little to drink, I made an appointment with the doctor. I remembered that her mother had gallstones at this age and had to have her gallbladder removed. I became more concerned that it might be something that couldn't be resolved at home with trial and error.

She got out of bed at about one (the appointment was at 3:30) and stumbled into the den holding her stomach in pain. I reminded her we were going to the doctor to find out what was wrong. "I have to take a shower," she proclaimed. I jumped on that, called the aide in from the other room, and started that process. Until Mom asked why she was taking a shower, and when reminded that she had asked for one, stated disdainfully, "I would never suggest such a thing in a million years!"

After some persuasion, they got the shower out of the way and got dressed. I had asked Marilyn to come with me to the doctor. Based on how weak Mom was acting and the pain she was in, I thought I'd have to go into the office for a wheelchair, and having someone to help me would be a good idea.

I pulled into a parking place and shifted the car into park. Mom hopped out of the car like she was ready to run a marathon. I checked us in with the receptionist and we took our seats in the waiting room. "Why are we here?" Mom kept asking.

In the examination room, Mom was equally baffled as to why she was seeing the doctor. As I listed her symptoms and painful episodes, she'd repeat, "Where was I?"

I tried to trick her into the truth but she was too clever for me. "If I came in with a bowl of ice cream right now, what would you say?"

For a week, she's said she couldn't eat it, she wasn't hungry, and her stomach hurt. Nope, she answered flatly that she'd say, "Thank you." I almost fell out of my chair.

The doctor, a round man with a patient bedside manor that she'd seen for years, said everything I'd done so far was what he'd suggest. His inclination was that acid reflux was the problem and to double her dosage of Prilosec. I also broke the 10mg Aricept in half and gave one in the morning and the other in the evening in case we were dealing with a side effect from her new prescription.

We returned home and Marilyn prepared a big bowl of ice cream to test her. Sure enough, she ate the whole thing. At night, I decided to act like she never had any problems with eating. I offered her chicken and rice or macaroni/tuna salad. She opted for the salad and ate a whole plate full. On the one hand, I was glad she ate. On the other hand, I felt like she'd been jerking me around. I'd been worried for over a week that she was going to die because I made an error in judgment, then we went to all the hassle of getting to the doctor, and she acted like I was the crazy one!

However, her discomfort returned, which led to an ultrasound at St. Mary's hospital looking for gallbladder issues and back to the doctor to have him tell us the results didn't show anything unusual.

Next step: I bought two sets of increasingly large underpants since she complained that what she was wearing hurt her stomach because they were too tight. I wondered if it could be that simple. Her underpants were too tight? "These hurt," she'd say, pulling at the waistband and releasing it with a snap.

What ended up solving the problem? Ex-Lax. That's right, she was constipated. Most likely due to dehydration. The doctor had asked about bowel movements during our office visit. I had heard her going to the bathroom just before we left the house so I told him there wasn't a problem. As her pain continued, I was more aware of monitoring her trips to the bathroom and her fluid intake.

Then I remembered something pertinent. She had stopped eating her daily bowl of oatmeal for breakfast. We had started that to keep her regular but she grew weary of eating it (can't say as I blame her) even though I bought every flavor under the sun. I started preparing Raisin Bran with sliced banana to keep her potassium levels up which had been low on one of her blood tests. That's when I think her digestive system got irregular.

It was back to oatmeal and some stool softener to prevent this from happening again. We had prescription Miralax and some

Metamucil to use on an ongoing basis.

As I've mentioned, dementia patients have a hard time identifying their ailments. In this case, severe stomach pain was as simple as constipation but it took us two trips to the doctor, once to the hospital, and two pair of underwear before we eventually figured it out. It was all necessary but it's a good illustration of how simple problems experienced by the elderly can be so expensive and taxing on the Medicare system.

* * *

She was aware that there was something really wrong with her mind. "Why don't they take X-rays or something?" I reminded her she'd been through all sorts of tests and countless doctors and specialists and that's why she took so much medicine. "What medicine," she demanded with an unbelieving tone like I was lying to her.

Then she asked if everyone knew that she "was like this." I told her that everyone that knows her knew that she'd been struggling with her health. That bothered her. Still a sense of vanity. Then she asked if her parents knew. I said they had died before this came on. "Good," she said with some satisfaction, and I knew it came from a place of not wanting to disappoint her family and add to their worries. We are a family of keeping things to ourselves. Push the emotions down, way down, and keep your mouth shut. There's always someone worse off and it's best to remember that before you start complaining.

* * *

I've heard that one of the stages of Alzheimer's is the increased use of profanity. There have been a couple of explanations for this. First is that there are "nasty" dementia patients who curse in conjunction with an overall rotten disposition. Second I've heard of Alzheimer's patients who swear out of frustration, namely when they can't remember something or know what they want to say but can't form the words to say it.

When we were getting ready to go for her bi-annual trip to the thyroid doctor, Mother Dear was looking for a washcloth. I reminded her that she had taken a shower the day before so that wasn't necessary. Marilyn had taken her to the beauty shop and she had her hair cut and permed. She told me, "I want to wash my face and ass." Okay, then! One washcloth, coming right up!

It was cold outside so I had Mom put on a fresh pair of undies, then thermal underwear, and a regular pair of pants on top. Close to the time we were heading out the door, she said her pants didn't fit. They looked fine to me, but she was clearly uncomfortable, and started to cry when she wanted to take them off and I was saying things were okay.

Into the bedroom we went to change out of those pants and into another. The problem was that she had gone to the bathroom before we left. She had forgotten to pull up her undies, only pulling up the long underwear and pants, so the undies were bunched up at her crotch. Once I figured out what was going on, we got things straightened out, and away we went.

* * *

Her knees were painful, one more swollen than the other, doubling the circumference of her leg. Her general practitioner diagnosed her with a Baker's cyst — accumulation of fluid in the knee joint. We were referred to an orthopedist to have it drained.

The orthopedist asked a series of questions to determine the cause of the inflammation and not just treat the symptom. Everything was checking out fine and he scratched his head, as he was deep in thought. He asked a final throwaway question:

Doctor: Do you live in an area where there are deer?

Bingo! Yes, we have deer in the back yard all the time and we have cats that bring ticks into the house. The official Lyme disease diagnosis came when the orthopedist ordered blood tests for gout and included the test for Lyme.

That was it. Lyme settles in the joints as it progresses after a couple of months so Mom had been infected for a while. There had been no telltale sign of a red bull's eye rash on the skin that anyone had seen so it went unnoticed and untreated. A bite from a Lyme disease-infected tick usually, but not always, results in a 2" red ring around the location where the tick had bitten.

That was our answer and she was put on a two-week dose of high-powered antibiotics. That left the fluid on the knee and what to do about it. The doctor put on gloves, sprayed the side of her leg with a freezing numbing agent, and inserted a long thick needle into the outer side of her knee. She jumped and screamed from the pain.

I held her down so the needle didn't accidentally poke something it wasn't supposed to when her leg recoiled in a jerking motion.

The specialist drained the knee and put in cortisone for some relief, which was very effective. She went from barely able to walk to climbing up the stairs with minimal effort when we got home. The procedure, however, was very painful.

We spent a Friday afternoon at her general practitioner for a follow up appointment for inflamed kidneys and the swollen knees. We'd spent months visiting her internist, a urologist, endocrinologist, and the orthopedist that originally drained the fluid from her knee. There were urine tests, blood tests, sonograms, a CAT scan, and a trip to the emergency room to figure out what was causing the severe pain in her side and back. Was it an infection? Nope, no sign of that. Was it kidney stones? There were traces of stones, but why were both kidneys inflamed at the same time and no evidence of a big stone?

As it turned out, the kidneys were inflamed as a side effect of a high dosage of Naproxen (Aleve) prescribed to lessen the pain and swelling she'd been experiencing in her knees before the Lyme diagnosis.

Her knee had accumulated more fluid so her regular doctor decided to drain it again and put in more cortisone while we were there. As I mentioned, this is a painful procedure even though they apply a topical freezing spray before they put the needle into the center of the knee. And this time was much worse than the previous time. This doctor went into the knee from the inside of the leg; the specialist went in from the outside, which may have been the difference.

This time she screamed, hollered, and cried. She jerked her leg while the needle was in it, which only made things worse. I had to hold her down on the examining table to keep her from doing any more damage. I whispered "Almost done" and "It'll be okay" in her ear but she was in no place to be consoled. It hurt, and we all knew her pain was real. The whole process only took about 10 seconds but it seemed like a lifetime. Even the doctor and nurse were all shook up.

She looked at me, betrayal in her watering eyes — I am supposed to be her protector and I had let her down. I had let these people hurt her with "the most excruciating pain I have ever felt." She declared she didn't trust any of us. The whole event then brought about a state of confusion where she didn't know where she was, who the doctor was, and why we were hurting her. She wanted to go home but was so weak and trembling she couldn't even stand. After calming down and taking a couple sips of water, we made our way home safe and sound.

I was to have tough decisions to make in the future. After this, she said she'd rather not walk than go through that again. But the knee was better. Would I put her through the pain again should it be required? Surely she would forget this episode by then and complain that no one was doing anything to help with her knee.

I was in the unfortunate position, with the advice of her doctors, to make those decisions.

* * *

It's not all without humor and rewards. When you ask a silly question, expect a silly answer. At a regularly scheduled doctor's appointment:

Doctor: So, how's your breathing?

Mom: I'm here, ain't I?

Both sides of the conversation were serious and I was the only one who laughed!

* * *

I had some pain in my lower back and I knew that I was going to pass a kidney stone. Kidney stone disease is hereditary. Mom had passed one in the hospital when I was little and I had inherited the disease in a big way. Mom's was made of calcium and she never drank milk or ate any dairy again.

I had a long history of them and recognized the symptoms right away. The pain went away but I was urinating quite a bit of blood a couple of days in a row. I hoped that the process would be easy although generally it was not. I'd had four surgeries and probably passed a dozen or more stones.

At 4 a.m., I started with pain in my left front side that radiated down to my family jewels. It continued to get worse and I began to pace in an effort to help it move. Mother Dear was asleep out on the couch so, after a while, I went in on her big bed and laid face down since that was the most comfortable position I could get in. Her routine had been to fall asleep in the den, wake up about 6 a.m. to go to the bathroom, and then go in to bed.

Mom came into the room and asked what was wrong and sat on the bed beside me. As I explained the pain from the stones, she started to gently rub my back. I thought that was sweet. Out of concern, she asked if I should contact a doctor. I told her no, that it would go away. Problem is that she kept asking the same line of questions about every five minutes. "Hello? Passing a kidney stone over here," I thought.

I eventually got up and took a Hydrocodone to quell the pain, she went to bed, and I fell asleep on the couch. My pain was gone but I knew that wouldn't last.

POOR ME

It had been a rough couple of weeks. I wasn't sure how much longer I would be able to take the pain in my back while managing to supervise my mother.

Passing kidney stones seemed to be about a three-month process for me — from the time I sensed something was wrong to the time I caught them in the strainer. This time was January to April.

It started as just a thought. I'd been feeling sick since mid-January. I thought it was depression, I thought it might be a sinus infection, I thought it might be a kidney stone getting ready to move. As it turned out, it was all three.

At the end of March, the pain began to escalate and I began passing blood in my urine. I had pain on the left side of my lower back. Not bad, but noticeable, and that's one of the first indicators of stone activity.

After a couple of days reprieve, the pain was back and I was up all night suffering. The spasms started about 10 p.m., and by midnight the cramps were so intense that they made me vomit. The stomach muscle is right next door to the kidneys and ureter and it got caught up in all the fun. I was awake for the next six hours — in between all the pacing. I had gone outside and walked up and down the street several times during the night. Walking helped to move the stone and provided some relief.

I finally couldn't stand the excruciating pain any more and went to the Emergency Room in the morning. But first I had to get coverage for Mother Dear. Luckily, Dan was close and able to skip out of work on an emergency basis. The pain had been intense for nine hours straight and the Hydrocodone pain medication wasn't even taking the edge off.

It was confirmed that I was passing a kidney stone although it didn't show up in either the KUB (Kidney, Ureter, and Bladder) X-ray or the ultrasound. Sometimes I psyched myself into thinking that maybe it was something much more dangerous like cancer, kidney disease, or a tumor. The only part of the ureter that wasn't visible in the ultrasound was the bottom portion hiding behind the bladder so that's where the stone must have been. That was good news because it had almost made it through the ureter, which is the painful part of its journey.

This all occurred on the left side. In the collection portion of the left kidney were two stones (8mm and 4mm) waiting to unleash. On the right, there was a 4mm in the kidney that was still a ways from leaving its womb.

I was given a new prescription for the more powerful Percocet painkiller. They found high levels of bacteria in my urine sample so I received the antibiotic Cipro. The spasms were really what caused me most of the pain and concern. I was given a prescription of Flomax for that.

After returning from the hospital, I continued with sporadic bouts of pain and bleeding. I learned that I was allergic to Percocet, causing me to have chills (my teeth were clacking they were chattering so hard), fever, and an itchy sensation over the lower half of my body.

I made an appointment with a new urologist to chart a course of action. He immediately suggested surgery, which made me suspect. Having been through this before, I considered that as the last option, not the first.

When the stone is in the ureter, the tube that runs from the kidney to the bladder, lithotripsy (shockwave therapy) requires the placement of a stent through the length of the ureter before the procedure. This allows urine to pass by the stone, thereby relieving the pain and preventing long-term damage to the kidney itself. The pain caused by a stone is the result of pressure placed on the kidney by a backup of urine that can't get by the stone. The stent allows the urine to pass the blockage.

The surgery option really meant two under-anesthesia operations and one office procedure. They go up through the urinary tract to place the stent in, the lithotripsy, and then taking the stent out at the doctor's office under local anesthetic.

When I refused to go through this (again), I was basically told to drink water and take the Percocet. I left the office after making the decision to tough it out.

During this time, Mom was trying to wander off while I was

dealing with the pain. I was angry and frustrated that I couldn't even have a sick day. Amidst a medical crisis, I still had to put her first because she couldn't and/or wouldn't behave.

She went outside to sweep the sidewalk and I went in and laid on the couch to rest because I hadn't slept for several nights. When Marilyn arrived, she found Mom lying semi-conscious in the backyard. She called the service provider, a nurse was dispatched, and I was grilled like I had been neglectful.

Two days later, I passed two 4mm stones.

Where did that leave me? The whole process wore me out. It drained me physically, mentally, and emotionally. And I knew I still had the 4mm within the right kidney, and a 4mm and an 8mm on the left that were closer to starting the passing process.

I felt the whole caregiving situation wasn't fair before, but this was the first time I really felt like it was a bad situation for me personally. When I had to find coverage before I could go to the Emergency Room, something was wrong, and I decided to place my needs higher.

I started looking for a nursing home. Over the years, I had tried to be sweet and nice to get Mom to do things but my patience had been exhausted. I had resorted to telling her that if she kept it up, she was going to require 24-hour care and that meant a nursing home. It wasn't nice to hold that over her head, but I didn't know what else to try even though she couldn't truly grasp the gravity of what I was saying.

Trying to be logical with a dementia patient isn't very logical at all. Of course, she couldn't remember a thing she had done so it was difficult to hold her accountable.

These threats did stay with her, afraid that we were plotting to put her away. She was right because something had to change.

III

THE DECISION

Traveling is the thing that gives me the greatest enjoyment. As I felt more and more burned out, I decided to get away. Getting out of the house by spending the afternoon at the Cineplex or shopping for groceries at the market just wasn't enough. Luckily, my brother was willing and able to take over mother sitting and spend overnights for a reasonable period of time. Planning vacations killed two birds with one stone — I was able to do what I loved most while restoring much of the energy I'd lost.

My first trip was to visit Melanie and Rick in Park City, just over the Wasatch mountain range from Salt Lake City. I've been fortunate to visit them at least a dozen times over the years. They have great hospitality from years of practice opening their home to friends and family. She calls it Hotel Mel. So many guests come and go they should install a revolving door!

In the winter, there's nothing like the snow at the Park City Ski Resort, which is the home of the U.S. ski team and was the site of some alpine events during the 2002 Winter Olympics. The bobsled and ski jump complex is not far away. The Sundance Film Festival is held there in January every year.

I was there in the summer and the highlight of the trip was a hike on the Mid-Mountain Trail that begins at the Silver Lake Lodge in Deer Valley and stretches through Park City to The Canyons and beyond. This is also known as the Eight Thousand Foot Trail because of its elevation above sea level. The air is thin, which makes mountain biking and hiking more challenging. There wasn't a cloud in the sky, it was warm, and there were abundant opportunities for me to take photos of the wildflowers along the trail. In short, it couldn't have been a more spectacular day. We made our way to the Red Pine Lodge for lunch, then doubled back to the car. As we hiked, mountain bikers zoomed past us on the dirt path.

The entire vacation was low key and there was a lot of time to decompress. Being in a situation away from home with friends gave me time to have some talks that I found therapeutic and renewed my perspective.

I was introduced to a lot of interesting new people at parties, restaurant gatherings, and my first Shabbat dinner. The week was perfect and just what I needed!

Next I paid a visit to my friend Rich in St. Petersburg. It was a bad omen when I felt light headed just after takeoff on the early morning departure flight. I was located in a middle seat and, by the time I decided I should wake up the person sitting on the aisle and get to the rest room, I fainted in my seat. I couldn't determine how long I was out but I woke up in a flop sweat feeling quite a bit better.

After arriving at my friend's place, I ended up spending practically the entire time curled up on the couch asleep and managing my stress belly. Seems I had traded the stress of caregiving for the worries of air travel, staying in a new place, and thinking about how things were going at the house. I made it a point to refrain from calling home because I wanted my time off to be a complete break. It would be a stretch to say I was a good houseguest. I was more of a house lump.

Rich was a great host and even better friend. He let me do what I needed. He didn't pry, no expectations, he was just supportive of me and where I was. I'm glad that he didn't take any time off from work because I would have felt guilty on top of the feelings of burn out.

During the days, I managed to get off the couch at about two in the afternoon and get out into the sunshine. It was chilly for Florida, but I was still able to get out for long walks with a jacket on. I meandered along the water of Coffee Pot Bayou, venturing on to enjoy the sight of palm trees, the beach, and the sun glimmering off the waves in Tampa Bay. I went out on the pier, made my way to downtown, checked out the stores, and then found a different route home where I could see the bungalows and tropical landscaping so common in the Historic Old Northeast neighborhood.

My host managed to get me out in the evenings for quick bites to eat. On Sunday it was over to the Gulf Coast to The Frog Pond restaurant in North Redington that was typically packed for brunch. Throw in a bit of shopping, more time on the beach, and the long weekend was a healthy dose of respite.

Six months later, I planned a weekend in New Orleans. I was at the end of my tether and the events in Florida seemed a distant memory. I had to get away, whether or not it was simply to sleep for a few days with a change of atmosphere. Jennifer had suggested we meet there and I jumped at the chance to escape again.

We searched online and found a charming bed-n-breakfast style inn called the Place D'Armes Hotel. The best feature was its location, location, location. Everything was within a short walking distance as it was in the heart of the French Quarter about a block from Jackson Square and St. Louis Cathedral. We had a stylish room but found it odd that there weren't any windows. That took a bit of getting used to.

I had more energy in Louisiana than Florida but my aching stomach had returned. I spent the weekend in New Orleans with my tummy in a tight ball, unable to eat much of anything. I wasn't able to completely relax and enjoy all of the high-end culinary delights for which the city is famous. When I was able to eat, we managed to try the French-style beignets at Café Du Monde with their café au lait blended with chicory, a couple of different po' boy sandwiches (a hero on light baguette-like bread), and a muffuletta (capicola, salami, pepperoni, ham, provolone and a marinated olive salad on focaccia-like bread).

There was so much to see walking around town. There was the boardwalk where I put in several laps, a lot of people selling original artwork, and the Steam Boat Natchez that called with a Saturday morning serenade on its powerful pipes. Perhaps the most interesting was the violin "playing" street musician with his instrument case open for donations. Except every time you walked by him, he was "tuning" the violin and never actually played anything. Quite a scam!

Bourbon Street was crowded but somehow more manageable sipping on rum-based hurricanes. Street musicians played there, a lot of nightclubs were open for business, and souvenir shops peddled Mardi Gras and voodoo trinkets.

With Jennifer's support and understanding, I did manage to catch up on my uninterrupted sleep and see enough of the city and its sights to know that I'd like to return someday.

You may be wondering: "I thought the whole point of taking the Paxil SSRI prescription was to eliminate the stomach aches." I was thinking the same thing. When I returned home, I made an appointment with the doctor and he decided to double the dosage. I'd been taking the pills for five years so it was likely that its potency had been diminished after prolonged use. Unfortunately, this higher amount exacerbated the constant ringing in my ears (tinnitus) to a level that made it impossible to fall asleep. If an angel gets its wings every time a bell rings, heaven was getting plenty full.

My appetite was still suppressed and I began to supplement what little I ate with nutritional Ensure drinks.

On a follow-up appointment with the doctor to express my concern about the tinnitus, he suggested a different prescription. It was the next-generation drug Lexapro that had a great track record with his other patients and showed few side effects. Unfortunately, the new medication made me feel much worse. I understood that it took a while for the body to adjust to anything new, especially something that is altering brain chemistry. I decided to stick with it in the hopes that things would get better as it took effect. That was a huge mistake.

Several weeks had passed when I had a terrifying medical incident. One afternoon, I experienced a blinding white headache so severe and unusual that it brought me to my knees. I began to think my time on good ol' planet Earth was coming to an early end.

I've never had a migraine headache so there was no point of reference. It was so bad that I thought it could be an aneurysm or stroke. I contemplated dialing 9-1-1 and making a trip to the emergency room in an ambulance but I waited to see if it would pass. The headache finally eased to a tolerable level about two hours later and I took two Ibuprofen. I had been reluctant to take anything right away because I didn't know what was wrong and many over-the-counter pain medicines can thin the blood. I was terrified that I might do something that could exacerbate the problem and bring about a tragic result.

I went back to the doctor the following day and conveyed the lack of progress on the new drug. I reported that I'd felt lousy since starting the prescription, like I was beginning to fall into an emotional hole. It clearly wasn't doing the job for which it was intended, so I was placed on yet another class of drug that was described as a "cleaner version" of the Paxil I'd been taking for years. The change to Pristiq resulted in an immediate improvement and I continued to take it without any side effects.

When I was feeling heightened anxiety, I had a supplemental prescription for the antihistamine that was successful over 30 years before that I could take as needed.

During the two-decade span of time after I had moved across the country, each doctor I saw insisted that the antihistamine I had taken in the 6th grade was an "old drug" and couldn't compare to the breakthroughs they'd made in the intervening years. My suggestions of, "If it ain't broke, don't fix it!" were always brushed aside with the assurance that the latest and greatest would be better. Now I'd come full circle and I was more confident than ever that I'd settled on the solution that worked for me. I learned to be more forceful in the decisions of my own medical care.

As for the headache that day, I was sent for an MRI on my brain to rule out that anything more serious was the cause. All the possible negative diagnoses ran wild through my mind. Was it indeed an aneurism or stroke? Maybe they'd find a tumor. Or worse. What could be worse? Who knows when it comes to the brain? Luckily the MRI showed that all things were normal. As normal as I'm ever going to be, as my friends would say, and a follow-up MRA showed there wasn't anything obvious by way of physical anomalies.

I'm still not sure what it was, but I'm pretty certain it was related to the new medicine and stress. The bottom line was that I was still burned out and I shouldn't be running back and forth to the doctor seeking relief from environmental conditions that needed to change.

The silver lining of the incident was that it brought a new clarity. It forced me to take a personal inventory of my life, consider where I was at and where my Mom was at. I needed to look seriously, honestly, and objectively at the entire situation. My mother could be like this for many years to come. Was I willing to live like this? For how long? Who defines what is reasonable? How is "quality of life" defined for my mother and me? At this rate, it felt like she was going to outlive me!

As with most things in my life, I had been waiting for a sign to provide me with the guidance I would need. As a young adult, I was full of plans and goals. Now, I'd become a procrastinator extraordinaire. I had considered that Mom might fall and break a hip, catch pneumonia, suffer a seizure or any other sort of major problem that would require her hospitalization. As terrible as that sounds, the difficult decision of what to do next would be taken out of my hands. Taking away the responsibility of making such a monumental decision would be a relief. However, rarely is life so clean that the solutions to complex problems come wrapped up in a pretty box with a brightly colored bow on top.

On reflection, my error was that I had been looking for direction from an external sign manifested by my mother. Indeed, I had been provided many signs, it's just that I hadn't been paying attention because they were coming in a way that I wasn't prepared to receive them. It finally occurred to me that the signs were happening *to* me and not *around* me. The knocking had been getting louder and it wasn't until I thought my own life was in danger did I open the door to new thinking. The realization hit me like a ton of bricks, providing an instant knowing of the way forward.

I simply had to save myself first.

After my epiphany, I spent many tearful conversations on the phone with Jennifer. I felt like I was caught between a rock and a hard place. On the verge of collapse, yet full of guilty feelings for not being able to handle more. I know it wasn't fair to me, but it didn't seem fair to Mother Dear either. She was going to suffer because I was weak.

I consulted with my brother and we decided to go ahead and place her in an assisted living home. The decision to place her was made quickly — all happening within a month — because I'd researched facilities a year earlier and decided where she would go when the time came. A perfect example of how forward planning can ease the amount of work that has to be done in a crisis.

I contacted the facility we chose and found out that a private room was available. It would be moving time after she received a final checkup and recommendation from her primary doctor, passed a state-mandated Tuberculosis test, and I had obtained a copy of her complete medical records.

The final doctor's appointment involved a general examination so he could fill out the required paperwork. He had to perform assessments of her mental and physical capabilities (or lack thereof) to verify that she would be able to function in the environment and administer the TB test. At the end of the exam, knowing what was happening, he asked her if she had any interest in going to live with other people her age. "No," Mom said gruffly. The doctor looked at me and shrugged. He thought he'd try to break the ice and make an official recommendation to her. Her response was no surprise to me because she'd told me she'd "run away" if anyone ever put her in such a place.

The move was going to be against her will. I'd say most elderly folks are initially against such a major upset to their lives. They are creatures of habit. Their surroundings and routines give them a feeling of familiarity and safety. Add dementia to the mix, where they already lack a sense of place and belonging, and they'd run for the hills if they had any choice in the matter.

Let's face it, there aren't many people, with dementia or otherwise, who want to be suddenly uprooted and live in an unfamiliar place with new sights, sounds, and strange people milling around.

For Mom, she was at the point where she didn't know where she was most of the time. I wasn't sure that being in a strange place would feel all that different to her. The move would provide her with the increased care that she now required, there would be plenty of activities specifically designed for someone in her condition, and she'd have the mental stimulation of interacting with more people. Being cooped up in the house isn't good for anyone. Me included!

I didn't know what to expect but I was sure we'd made the correct decision. A sense of relief washed over me like a warm shower although there was still a lot of sadness and fear of what lied ahead. What the future held for her, and what the future held for me. I had a bundle of personal concerns. I'd held the position of caregiver for four years and the prospect of reinventing myself and starting life over was a bit daunting. Possibilities included a new job, new place to live, and even travel.

Another crucial factor that contributed to this rather sudden decision was that Marilyn was scheduling surgery to repair a disintegrating disc in her neck. She expected to be out for several months and I wasn't very confident that she would ever be able to come back.

There was the option of having the agency send other aides but I wasn't prepared to deal with that. The jobs are low pay and generally thankless so many of the people who take these positions, or the ones that the agencies can find to fill them, are notoriously unreliable. The gem we had was irreplaceable with her level of loyalty, professionalism, reliability, trustworthiness, and the comfort level she had with our family.

All I knew was that I was burned out; suffering from the physical effects of stress, and couldn't continue with things as they were.

The decision was made. It was best for her, best for me, and best for all of us.

FACILITIES

When it became increasingly evident that keeping Mom at home was untenable, which turned out to be about a year before her eventual move, I began to evaluate places where Mom could go that were comfortable, pleasant, safe, and affordable.

I discovered there are about as many types of facilities as there are facilities themselves. Most try to carve out a unique niche in the market that makes them more desirable than the next. In the past, our society referred to them as "rest homes," "retirement homes" or "old folks' homes." Then "nursing homes" became the catchall term. For the sake of simplicity in the following descriptions of on-site visits, I've narrowed it down with my own description of four general categories.

Independent Living: These are individual apartments or condominiums set aside specifically for senior citizens only. Residents require no outside assistance and, as the term implies, they are capable of living independently. They may or may not have cafeterias or common eating areas where meals can be purchased. Larger developments may have recreational areas such as bocce ball courts, horseshoe pits, or even golf courses. Transportation to supermarkets and malls may also be provided.

Assisted Living: The residents are high functioning and many are able to get around independently with or without assistance of a device such as a cane, walker, or wheel chair. These facilities provide meals, on-site nursing staff, bathing assistance, dispensing of medication, transportation services to doctors' appointments, and field trips.

Assisted Living with Memory Care: A subset of Assisted Living, these are a concept specifically designed for patients suffering from some form of dementia or memory loss. Residents may or may not have physical disabilities in addition to their mental incapacity.

Nursing Home: These facilities provide a very high level of care for those that aren't able to get around on their own, need assistance getting out of bed, or are bedridden. Physical rehabilitation is usually offered to overcome the debilitating physical ramifications of a health crisis. These could be the result of surgery such as a hip or knee replacement, broken bones from a fall, or more systemic problems such as those experienced after a stroke.

My research began by asking friends and neighbors for recommendations. Word of mouth gets past the colorful brochures and slick sales pitches. I did some research on the Internet and reviewed the web sites of places in the area with sterling reputations. After narrowing it down to five places, I scheduled an appointment for a tour at each location.

Before I even made it to any of the sites, I played out the worst-case scenarios in my mind. Every site was going to be a horror with people drugged up in hospital beds, moaning and screaming, clutching at my clothes and begging me to help them escape. Surely I was going to be transported straight into the throes of Ken Kesey's *One Flew Over the Cuckoo's Nest*. There would be tile floors with a high shine, flickering fluorescent light fixtures atop long nondescript corridors, walls painted in battleship gray and doors with frosted glass letting in a minimum of filtered light. Anonymous nurses, donned with knee length white dresses and navy cardigan sweaters, would walk smartly from room to room as the rubber souls of their white shoes squeaked with every stride.

My imagination churned up a plethora of scary possibilities that ended up being nothing like what I actually encountered.

Location #1

Location 1 clearly put those preconceived notions to rest. The site was a combination Assisted Living/Assisted Living with Memory Care facility. It felt like I was approaching a modern luxury hotel when I drove up to park the car and I half expected to be greeted by a bellman at the front door.

The building was new construction with neatly trimmed foundation shrubs and colorful flowers that lined the sidewalk. Residents were on the front porch sitting on benches to enjoy the beautiful summer day. They nodded or said "hello" as I passed.

The four-star feeling continued as I passed them and was warmly greeted upon my entry by a perky gal behind the reception desk. On the counter in front of her was a nicely formatted menu of the meals for the day. This was one of the many nice touches I noticed throughout the visit. Every meal featured a few new daily entrees that supplemented the everyday grill selections of hamburgers, hot dogs, and sandwiches that were always available.

The receptionist asked my name, placed a call to the account manager who would be my tour guide, and asked me to wait in the seating area behind me. The waiting area was a library with a large selection of books that filled a custom-built floor-to-ceiling bookcase constructed of dark stained wood. The books were available to the residents and most appeared to have been donated by the residents themselves — probably when they sold their homes and relocated. What to do with all of their perfectly good books? Bring 'em to the new place so everyone can enjoy them!

Angela, the account manager, emerged from her office. She met me with a handshake and a smile that foretold of her bubbly personality. She was clearly cut out for a sales position and we got along incredibly well.

She explained that there were two levels of assisted living within the single building where we stood. There were about 50 residents on the current floor; 16 residents, all women, were on a level below in the memory care area.

After she explained everything on the main floor, we went to an elevator that took us down to the memory care area. It was completely separate from the people living above. Entering a password on a keypad was the only way to activate the elevator. This was the mechanism in place to prevent residents in this section from leaving the floor and possibly wandering away.

As we descended, I was warned that it was all women and a few of them were known to be a bit frisky. Seeing a man could generate an uncomfortable situation. Sure enough, one woman nearly tripped over herself when we emerged from the elevator. In no time, she had her hand on my shoulder and was asking if I was single. She had goosed a prior tour taker so the physical expression of her romantic intentions towards me could have been much worse.

Despite being on the lower level, it was not a basement, and all of the rooms had full windows and their own shower. There was access to a beautifully kept enclosed courtyard from the lobby area located next to the dining room. Meals were served at the same time every day with a fixed seating plan. The attendants on duty would find everyone and get each to their assigned place.

I happened to be there mid-afternoon, right at the beginning of sundowner's syndrome, so all of the patients had been gathered in the activities room to be led through a game. Mental stimulation is commonly used to redirect attention.

This site was a single location of a national chain of for-profit facilities. The cost was around $5,600 per month. Items like hair appointments, manicures and pedicures, and transportation to a doctor or medical facility were provided at an additional cost. If the resident ran out of money and was unable to maintain their monthly payments, they would be given 30 days notice.

Location #2
Location 2 was a Nursing Home where the worst part of the aging process practically rose up out of its bed and slugged me square across the jaw. It was here that I experienced many of the preconceived notions that I had feared. Most of the residents were bedridden; some were parked in wheel chairs just outside of their rooms and were either asleep or seemed drugged. I didn't see anyone walking around except for the staff and a few visitors. This seemed to be a place where people came for the countdown to death.

In my description here, I don't mean to denigrate nursing homes in any way. They provide a crucial and much needed service in the most compassionate way they can. Anyone who works with the elderly has to be a special person in order to deal with it on a daily basis.

There wasn't much for my tour guide to show me. Decor was sparse; the entire building felt bright and airy. There was a simple dining area, small in size because most meals were served in bed.

A "rehabilitation center" had a few pieces of exercise equipment and I made a mental note that the apparatus wasn't worthy of being in a home gym. I stopped myself with that thought. The observation taught me that I needed to recalibrate my expectations during the evaluation process. It's important to judge things appropriately based on the needs of the patient rather than what one would find in the world at large. When I caught myself looking for the rows of elliptical machines and weight benches, I had to take a step back and realize that most of the people there couldn't stand up let alone walk on a treadmill. What was I expecting? Spin classes and Pilates?

If a patient was in need of specific rehabilitation, inspecting this area and speaking with the physical therapist would be a good idea.

Ask about their education and training. What would be a sample exercise plan? In their experience, what was the time frame for a patient to recover from various maladies?

As for wandering, the receptionist at the front desk was the only prevention. I suppose security needs are minimal when most patients aren't going anywhere and the others were barely mobile.

This location was locally run and the cost was about $290 per day. Nursing homes are higher priced because the staff is required to provide a higher level of care. In most Long Term Care insurance policies, nursing homes qualify for an elevated tier of reimbursement, as their charges are commensurately higher.

At the outset of my tours, I thought that my mother would be in a Nursing Home. Once I started the tours, I realized that there were a lot of folks in much worse condition than she was and further visits to Nursing Homes weren't required. I needed to focus on assisted living centers with some form of memory care from that point forward. A nursing home would be a step further down the road.

Location #3

Location 3 was adjacent to Location 2. They were next-door neighbors but unaffiliated. It was an Assisted Living facility where residents with and without dementia shared a common space. The building was nice and grounds neatly kept. A long burgundy awning covered the sidewalk and there was a bench alongside as I approached the entrance. I pushed open the glass front door and smelled that distinct hospital odor of disinfectant. It's a smell you notice immediately but become accustomed to almost as fast.

The entrance to the building opened into a hallway, not the lobby, which I thought was an unusual layout. I later learned that the original part of the building had been a hen house, which was converted into the administration area.

There was a clear oval vase atop a glass table with a stem of silk phalaenopsis orchids placed inside. There was solidified acrylic made to look like water that kept the stem in place. To the immediate right was a large activities room where many were gathered to watch the big screen television and partake in activities such as Bingo and sing-a-longs. It was the first day of a new recreation director and he seemed a bit flustered as he darted around like a busy bee. I turned left and there were two offices, one on each side of the hall. On the left were the nurses in charge of medical care. The account and administrative staffs were in the office on the right where management, billing, and related tasks were handled.

I gently knocked on the door and announced myself to the account staff. I met briefly with them to discuss some general financial questions before beginning the tour. Rosemary, the nurse in charge of the floor staff and responsible for the overall care of the residents, was my guide. While I don't think she told me anything that any other person wouldn't have, it was nice to get a feel for the person that was in charge and hands-on with the residents and not a salesperson trying to sell me the next available bed.

As we walked through the various corridors, I noticed things were a bit downscale from Location 1. Instead of chandeliers there were light fixtures. Rather than fancy wallpaper, there was paint. In place of napkins and place mats made of cloth, they had paper.

On a side note here, and to acknowledge how little things can have an effect on the ultimate decision, the paper place settings in the dining room had pictures and brief descriptions of wild birds. I asked if I could have one and took it home to show my mother because she liked everything associated with wildlife. I used a magnet to affix it to the front of the refrigerator. I also asked myself, "What is more important to Mom: plain cloth placemats or something interesting to look at that happens to be made of paper?"

The lobby was central to the building's layout and the epicenter of activity. The main nurses' station was located there with a panel of lights that signaled when an upstairs resident needed assistance. The medication cart and schedules for what aide was to assist which resident were also here. In this way, too, it seemed more like a hospital setting.

Many residents were sitting on sofas and chairs positioned against the walls around the room, watching the goings-on and looking out onto an enclosed courtyard planted with Tamarack trees, evergreens, shrubs, and annual flowers. People were in their wheelchairs and seemed happy to be out in the hub of activity. Some folks were outside on the large cement patio in the center of the courtyard. Several porch swings were strategically placed so the aides could keep a close watch through the oversized windows that were framed by heavy burgundy drapes.

The dining room was decorated with a country theme and country music was playing from a CD spinning in a player mounted vertically on the wall. Teal fabric cushions were tied on the oak chairs' seats with six per table. There were two shifts for dinner and everyone had an assigned time and seat. Aides would locate the various residents and bring them to the dining room where they would be seated. All residents were expected to eat with the group and meals were only served to a few residents in their rooms. Afternoon medications were also dispensed at this time.

There were no menus or selections; everyone was served the same modest meal with a choice of sugar-free soda, lemonade, coffee, tea, or water to drink. The menu was written in ink on a dry erase board. Those that needed extra nutrients or were losing weight were given high-calorie protein shakes in small school-sized milk cartons. They had a similar formula to those that can be purchased in a grocery or drug store.

The building had two wings on the ground floor with about 20 rooms each and a wing upstairs with 12 rooms that were accessible by an elevator or stairs. Most had their own bathroom and could be configured to be a private or double room. There were bird cages throughout with two parakeets apiece that chirped away.

There was a real assortment of people living there. Some with physical ailments and others with mental disorders. From 60 years old to 100+. Primarily women with a fair representation of men. Bracelets worn by at-risk patients activated sensors at all exits to control wandering.

The place was for-profit and run by a local company. The cost was $128 per day (~$4,000 per month) for a private room and services such as hair appointments and transportation to a doctor or a medical facility were a nominal fee. Manicures were done free-of-charge by the activities staff. However, only a podiatrist was allowed to trim toenails on monthly visits. (I think this was a state health regulation.)

If a resident ran out of money, they would be given 30 days notice.

Locations #4 & #5
Locations 4 and 5 were run by the same local not-for-profit organization with a great reputation in elder care. Location 4 was their first facility specifically designed and constructed for dementia patients. Location 5, about 30 miles south of its predecessor, took the same basic idea and floor plan and added some minor tweaks they discovered during Location 4's operation. There were only woman residing at Location 4 while Location 5 was 20 percent men.

Several buildings were on the property of Location 5. Some were for Independent Living, some for Assisted Living, and one was

Assisted Living with Memory Care. The feeling was very much like an expensive hotel and comparable to Location 1. I asked my guide when I could move in!

The entrance opened to a large lobby that looked like a mountain lodge with high ceilings and a lot of lightly colored pine paneling. Magazines were placed on coffee tables in front of overstuffed sofas in the waiting area and the hum from a fish tank filter filled the otherwise silent air. I checked in with the receptionist who summoned the account manager with a phone call to announce my arrival.

Randi met me with a broad smile, presented me with some literature, and guided me to a short hallway off the corner of the lobby. It led to a door with a security lock. After entering the code, we proceeded through to another world. I found myself in a place that no one except the residents, staff, and those privileged with the magic door code would ever see. The space kept a certain segment of our community safely locked behind a heavy door to protect them from society — and society from them.

The building was arranged with a floor plan based on pods. There were three pods connected at the center and each had twenty rooms, a common seating area with a large screen television, and a kitchen accessible to all. There were several alcoves along the corridors with floor-to-ceiling windows where residents were sitting and chatting amongst themselves.

A large outdoor area was accessible to everyone as well. It was enclosed with a high fence and featured a circular sidewalk to keep residents from getting lost. If they started out on the path, it would lead them through the yard and right back to the door where they could come back in. All paths led home. Swings and chairs were located along the walk for anyone that wanted to take advantage of nice weather and get a breath of fresh air.

I was impressed that all of the patients seemed to recognize my guide and genuinely like her. She told me she'd taken an extended absence to have a baby and that her toddler was a big hit whenever she brought her in to work. Elderly people seem to love babies!

Meals were handled in a much different way from what I'd previously observed. There was no fixed seating or dinnertime. Residents were encouraged to live their lives at their own pace and they were permitted to eat whenever they were hungry. I'm still not sure how this played out in reality since people like my mother had to be told what and when to eat. They couldn't remember it was dinnertime, usually didn't feel hungry, and lacked the ability to make a selection from multiple choices provided to them. Mom did much better when told exactly what, where, and when to eat.

A special room holding many stations of mentally stimulating activities was along the tour but there wasn't anyone using any of it at the time. There was a baby doll that needed tending to, washcloths to be folded, and beads to be pushed from one end to the other along a wire with an intricately curved path.

The price of about $5,600 per month was reflected in the expensive level of the property's accoutrements. Items like hair appointments, manicures and pedicures, and transportation to a doctor or a medical facility were additional costs. A financial analysis before acceptance would determine admittance. Once a resident was admitted, they were there for life regardless if they ran out of money.

A year passed between the time I did my homework and when it was time to place my mother.

My brother and I opted for Location 3 for several reasons. The staff and facility came highly recommended by friends who had relatives there. The facilities were a bit below the others, but the cost was also $1,600 less per month. Those items that weren't as nice were important to me yet wouldn't make any difference in the long-term health and safety of our mother. After all, the color of the carpet, the dinner placemats, and the wallpaper weren't as important as long as they were clean.

Location was also paramount in our decision. It was in Hoosick Falls where my mother had spent much of her time growing up and living there would place her near family and older friends. Given her age, there was a high probability that childhood friends and schoolmates, distant relatives, and acquaintances from this small town would also be there to provide her with an established base of friends.

After making our decision, I spoke with a close friend who placed his mother in an expensive facility that had all the bells and whistles. Her level of care escalated as her physical health declined after she was admitted. The facility deemed that she needed around-the-clock care and began exorbitant supplemental charges for the extra coverage. I learned that this should have been on my standard list of questions to ask during the interviews.

Their family ended up going with an unconventional solution. The friend's father began to require a higher level of care, which would have meant twice the expenses for two people in assisted living. The family sold their house, rented a two-bedroom apartment in a brand-new community, and hired a full-time caregiver to live with the couple. She was provided room, board, and a salary — she was happy for the opportunity.

I had considered this, going so far as to meet with their caregiver to get a sense of how such a situation might work. I decided against it because I would still be living in the house with my mother and I wasn't sure about taking on another person to live with. Who would take care of the caregiver when they were sick in bed with the flu? Who would be financially responsible if they needed to go to the hospital? I envisioned scenarios where I could end up taking care of two people instead of just the one. I was looking for help, not more responsibility!

Lastly is something that can never really be known ahead of time but bears mentioning. What are the other residents like? After the move, I visited my mother regularly, raising my consciousness that this was close-quarters communal living. The residents live together, eat together, relax together, exercise together, watch television together, and play games together. They spend all their time within the confines of the same perimeter walls. Whether someone will get along with the others is anyone's guess and it's probably the most important thing of all.

I'M SORRY, MOTHER DEAR

My brother and I approached the big day with a lot of trepidation. In retrospect, it went rather smoothly and we did a great job remaining calm and keeping our own emotions in check. It wasn't until I returned home to an empty house that I broke down and sobbed.

We had agreed ahead of time that we would tell my mother a story about how we'd found a new specialist that was going to help her with her memory. For the month prior to the move, every time she would complain about her lack of memory or become frustrated from a loss for words, I would remind her that we were going to change doctors to see if there was anything a new specialist could do. I was hoping that the seed would be planted and grow within her memory with continued watering of the subject. Unfortunately for her and millions of others with Alzheimer's and other forms of dementia, there is no cure or real hope.

My brother came up with a brilliant idea that she would be "admitted to the hospital for tests" so the doctors could evaluate her condition. There was a kernel of truth to it and she went along with optimistic hope. She would have resisted an assisted living center if we'd been direct about it but recent history showed that she had no such fear of hospitals. It was a lie, yes, but one that benefitted everyone, including her.

I packed some of her clothes into two paper shopping bags the weekend before the move. If she saw a suitcase, I was convinced she would ask questions and it would cast doubt on the story we were crafting. I think that was my own paranoia. It's doubtful she would have noticed a suitcase let alone understood that it was for her and what that might indicate. When my brother arrived the following Monday morning, Mom was still in bed so we moved the bags to his car's trunk without her knowing.

She awoke when she heard his voice and we continued to treat things as if it was a normal day and he was paying a regular visit. Mom made her way out of the bedroom, shuffled down the hall, through the kitchen, and plopped down on the couch in the breezeway. I poured a glass of orange juice and prepared her pills like I did every other morning. After she gulped them down, we stated matter-of-factly that we were going to see the special memory doctor as soon as we could all get ready. She took it in stride, which was not quite what I had expected. I kept waiting for her to catch on.

I began to get her ready to go. While I washed her hair in the sink, I thought about how it was going to be the last time I'd be doing it and was mindful to enjoy the experience. Mundane tasks can be special when it becomes the last time you'll do them. I took out a fresh set of comfortable clothes and helped her change into them. Then it was out to the car and away we went.

It was an unsettling half-hour journey. My mind raced and I squirmed in my seat the entire time. On the bright side, it was a beautiful drive and the summer weather couldn't have been more beautiful. It was sunny and warm with no humidity. The fields were green, rolling hills dotted with black-and-white Holstein dairy cows in the distance, and the rows of corn were high and preparing to tassel already. The road wound through Tibbits National Forest where the trees stood stoically alongside as if they'd seen it all before, maintaining a sereneness that conveyed, "This too shall pass." A brook babbled alongside the road, making its way along the lowest part of the mountain pass that had been carved by a glacier and revealed as the ice age came to an end.

The car was silent except for the radio that was tuned to an easy listening station and the volume was turned down as to be hardly audible.

Afterwards, my brother and I discussed the trip and he said something that I had also thought. For him, it felt like the time he took his ailing dog for her last walk before putting her to sleep. I, too, had a similar feeling. Like when I put down my cat after 16 years due to inoperable liver cancer. It crossed my mind that our journey with Mom was a bit like leading an innocent lamb to slaughter. I thought of Francesca, her lamb that disappeared when she was little.

Mom was in such a place mentally that she was going along without a clue of what lied at the end of the leisurely ride. While not death, she was going to a place where she had repeatedly said she never wanted to go. And here were her two boys, literally entrusted with her life with Power of Attorney and Do Not Resuscitate paperwork in hand, pulling a fast one on her.

It seems a bit dramatic but a lot of conflicting things go through one's mind. I knew it needed to be done. The way we did it was for the best, as it caused no distress in her. The staff had been told of the hospital story ahead of time so they knew what to expect and to keep from contradicting anything we might say. They warned us it is usually harder on the family than the person. I'm not sure that ended up being the case, not knowing first hand how my mother felt, but I can affirm that it sure wasn't easy for us.

When we arrived, my brother dropped us off at the front door and then went to park the car. I took a hold of her hand for reassurance and we started up the sidewalk. I commented about how nicely the landscaping was maintained and she pointed at the pretty begonias with delicate pink flowers and purple leaves.

We entered, passing the activities room that was full of residents. Mom asked, "Did you see all the old people in there?" I nodded my head in the affirmative and proceeded directly to the administrator's office where I made a quick round of introductions.

My brother caught up to us when we were already heading to her room. Once we were seated in the chairs and on the bed, I told her that this was going to be her hospital room since the doctors wanted her to stay for observation and tests. I thought this was when the light bulb was going to go on, that we were going to leave her behind in an old folk's home, but it didn't.

The supervising nurse on duty, the same one who had given me the original tour of the place a year before, asked Mother Dear if she would like to go for a walk. "Yes," Mom said with a smile, enjoying the special attention. Out they went, hand in hand, and down the hall as she was given a tour of the place. My brother and I scurried out to the car and got her things, ran back to her room, and unpacked three bags. Mostly clothes, with some bathroom items like her toothbrush, a bar of soap, shampoo, and deodorant.

I'd also packed her stuffed polar bear. It was wearing a white sweater with "Hug Me" knitted in a big red heart across its chest. Fuzzy Butt the bear stared blankly forward when I sat him on her pillow with his back leaning against the headboard. In that way, I imagined that Mother Dear and the bear were going to spend an extraordinary amount of time in bed together doing the same thing.

Next stop was the nurses' station to complete the final paperwork, tie up loose ends, and deliver the remaining pills from prescriptions that had been filled when she was still at home. We explained again what she liked and didn't like. Ice cream was a sure fire hit when all else failed. Of basic flavors, coffee was preferable, but hot fudge sundaes with vanilla ice cream were winners, too.

By the time we left, she was sitting in the activities room with everyone else. We learned that Theresa, an Activities Director, was from the area. She knew all of my mother's history and our extended family. She adopted Mom as her new best friend in order to help her adjust to the unfamiliar people and surroundings.

As mentioned, a main consideration in choosing this particular place was the hope that she might find people that knew her. Our thinking had paid off on the first day within the very first hour. They were sitting together and chatting like old friends right from the start.

I asked my brother if he thought we should go in and say "Goodbye." His answer was a quick "No." I asked, "Is that for her benefit or yours?" He replied, "Both." I respected that answer given that Mom was already settling in and she wouldn't remember us leaving anyway. For the sake of a smoother transition we opted to leave discreetly rather than cause a scene.

We were advised to stay away for a couple of weeks because it would help her adjust.

And that was that. On our drive home, Dan said, "Today is the day I've dreaded for eight years."

There were no tears until I walked in the door at home. It was a bit like experiencing a death. Emotions burst forth and I started crying and found myself repeating, "I'm sorry. I'm so sorry."

- I'm sorry you have this terrible disease. A disease that steals your personality. Your memories. Your sense of space and belonging. Your knowledge. It stole your golden years. It stole your retirement. It reached back through the years and stole your entire life.

- I'm sorry that I couldn't hold out any longer. That my personal health was such that I couldn't keep you comfortably at home.

- I'm sorry that you'll never come home to this house where you lived for so long and it had served you so well.

Where you spent 60 years of your life, 38 of them with your husband, and raised two children.

- I'm sorry you'll no longer be able to see your yard where you gardened endlessly to keep the flowers blooming, the vegetables growing, the grass green, the leaves raked, and the weeds at bay.

- I'm sorry that you will never have the loving companionship of the two cats that greeted me at the door when I got home.

The first 24 hours I spent alone in the house were really tough. Some memories caused me to sob. Other thoughts weren't as upsetting and simply brought tears welling up in my eyes. She would never come home again. Everything reminded me of her. She had decorated the home with prized possessions and purchased each piece of furniture. Her personality reached out from every item lovingly hung on the walls, placed on the counters, and displayed in curio cabinets.

The interesting emotion that crossed my mind was guilt. Guilt for the normal reasons, yes, but also for one I hadn't expected. There I was, in her house, enjoying her things after I had put her in a place where she couldn't. It felt like I had stolen everything from her.

All in all, I think the day of separation went well for her considering what actually happened. I cried most of the day.

* * *

Old habits die hard. For weeks after I first started living alone again, much of what I did and thought seemed to be a strange innate behavior. The routine with my mother had been practiced so much it was without thought.

When I would leave the house to run errands I found myself in a hurry because my subconscious instructed me to return home to Mom as quickly as possible. I was conditioned that the aide was going to leave at five o'clock and being back on time was the highest priority.

Other times, I would wake up and catch myself listening for sounds of movement to detect if Mom was awake yet. Now that she was living somewhere else, she'd probably been up and had breakfast already — just in a different place.

I discovered that Mother Dear had become a convenient excuse for my own shortcomings. I caught myself blaming her when I couldn't find my reading glasses. "My glasses. Where the hell are my glasses?" I repeated to myself over and over. Then my mind went to Mom and wondered where she'd "hidden" or misplaced them. Except she wasn't around. Damn!

Autumn came quickly and was in full stride. The leaves were dropping from our trees both front and back, each colorful leaf floating delicately to the grass below. They quickly accumulated to form a crinkly beige carpet that crunched under foot. Mother Dear loved to watch me rake up the leaves during the fall.

The first year of my return I had hurt my back holding up a gas-powered blower in an effort to corral the leaves. I'd blow them into a pile, put on the vacuum attachment, and grind them up as they were sucked into the bag. The weight of the blower and a full bag of leaves put my lower back muscles into such tight spasms that I couldn't move the next day. Those muscles are still sensitive to any sort of extended strain.

The following year I borrowed a lawn mower from my brother and ground up the leaves into smaller pieces. I raked the shreds into compact piles, placed them into large brown Kraft bags, and put them by the roadside for pickup. That was easier on my body but proved to be inefficient.

Finally, the next year, I borrowed my neighbor's lawn mower with a bag attachment. It didn't hold a whole lot but it was more efficient and less taxing than the other means I had tried.

As I mowed and bagged, I'd catch myself scanning the windows along the back of the house for my mother. She either sat in the rocking chair and watched, or stood and looked out the kitchen window to monitor my progress. She always smiled and waved excitedly when my eyes caught hers.

It didn't hit me when I first looked to the breezeway and she wasn't sitting in the chair. I shifted my eyes to the kitchen figuring I would find her watching me from there. Then it struck me anew that she wasn't there anymore, and as corny as it sounds, tears rolled down my cheeks. Again, one of those mindless tasks we do that take on a heightened level of meaning when you realize it will be the last experience of its kind.

She would never watch me rake the leaves again. Everything could have turned into such a memory — I'll never experience that with her again — but only certain things triggered those thoughts. Most of them mundane.

* * *

The stress that I had felt as a caregiver didn't lift right away. I had expected to immediately feel like a ton of bricks had been lifted from my shoulders. Instead, I found myself worrying for a different reason. I had been feeling the crush of responsibility on a 24/7 basis. That commitment gave way to the guilt of not being able to watch over her 24/7 and protect her.

My own physical and mental health began to improve about a month later. I started to feel better with my spirits lifting as the depression waned. My eating habits improved as my stomach aches subsided.

The feelings of dread were replaced by an increase in energy and a better outlook on life. I began to sleep uninterrupted through the night, which lead to more energy during the day. I cleaned. I organized. I gardened. I had been conditioned to feel defeated and burned out and the change helped me turn the corner.

The necessary steps had been taken to solve a desperate situation.

A GOOD DAY OR A BAD DAY

The first time I saw my mother after the initial drop off, I took her to meet her new doctor. It made sense to reconsider her primary care physician with the change of location. Based on a recommendation from the staff, we selected a local general practitioner who also served as the medical director of the care facility. His offices were a few blocks away which meant easy transport should she need to go. He already had a working relationship with the nurses and was completely aware of their procedures.

The first appointment was important. The transportation manager could have taken her but it was their first meeting. I wanted to take advantage of the consultation to fill him in on her extensive medical history while it was still fresh in my mind. I could recite all of the doctors she'd seen, what they had said, and the reasons for her various prescriptions. I was also interested in sizing him up.

I was a bit worried that Mom would think I'd come to take her home but she was fine the entire time. No need to use any of the excuses I'd invented ahead of time. She was a bit zombie-like but she knew whom I was when the doctor asked, as part of his interview, to determine where she stood from a mental standpoint.

After his evaluation was complete, he said matter-of-factly that her memory was shot. The bluntness, especially in front of her, made me uneasy — I knew it was the case but it still didn't feel good to actually hear someone else say it out loud. It's a bit like hearing someone say your sister is ugly. It's okay for you to say it but an entirely different thing for anyone else to say it.

The doctor said that a recent study questioned the affectivity of the Alzheimer's drugs she was taking to restore her memory or at least slow the downward trend of memory loss. We agreed to continue on with them since there was no way of knowing if removing them from her daily regimen would have a negative effect. The restoration of her memories was beyond any hope at this point.

I saw her on Independence Day and it didn't go as well. I found her standing in the lobby crying when I walked in. I hugged her and asked what was wrong. She was discombobulated, her mind going in all directions until she told me that someone had pulled her hair. It was difficult to get a coherent explanation out of her so I reported it to the staff. It could have been a staff member as she said, another resident, or just in her mind. I didn't know, and unless someone saw it happen, there was no way to ever really know for sure. As the saying goes, if I knew then what I know now, I wouldn't have gotten angry. If indeed it had happened as she said, it could have been any one of the many residents wandering around with dementia and likely a random event.

I took her by the hand and led her to her room. She resisted my efforts to get her to relax on the bed and take a nap. No amount of reasoning resonated with her. Full of energy, with adrenaline still pumping, she asked me to walk the halls with her. We ended up on a courtyard swing until it was time to eat.

My brother and I had worked into a routine for visiting. We strategically arrived about an hour before dinnertime. That way we had the opportunity to leave without any fanfare while her attention shifted to the dining experience. There was a lot for her to pay attention to: going to the bathroom first, getting to the dining room, sitting in her assigned spot, saying "hello" to her table mates, and then on to drinks and eating. Making any inkling that we were leaving or saying goodbye generated tears on her part. A simple, "I'll be back" as we left seemed to work best.

A problem during her adjustment period was her lack of hunger. She would resist efforts to get her seated in the dining room. We tried to redirect her thoughts over and over to keep her on track without much success.

On this day, she was still observably agitated and it could have been related back to the earlier incident. An attendant saw me struggling and tried to help with no success.

Me: Why don't you follow me? Let's go into the other room.

Mom: [Angry.] I'm not going anywhere with you!

Me: Why? What's the matter?

Mom: [Wild eyed with a raised voice.] Because you're always mean to me!

I looked at the attendant, she looked at me, and we shrugged simultaneously. As quickly as Mom got angry, she moved on to her normal mood. I considered that she might have thought I was the "hair puller." I eventually got her to her seat in the dining room and scooted out when they served her vegetable soup and a ham sandwich.

* * *

A few days later I received a call from the nurse. She expressed concern that Mom was continuing to have trouble adjusting. She seemed nervous and was crying a lot. I agreed, recounting how I had found her crying earlier in the week. They had put her on the protein shakes to address weight loss from not eating, and the nurse suggested that we increase her anti-anxiety medication.

We agreed to an increase if it was going to help. I had considered mentioning the same thing to the nursing staff. It was a great decision because she clearly became calmer. It was still a bit of a wrestling match to get her in for dinner but she was less tearful. Her appetite returned and she eventually put on enough weight to warrant new pants that were two sizes larger!

* * *

Shortly after the initial move-in, I brought two vases and a couple of house plants to place on her windowsill given that gardening and flowers were always a passion of hers. The first was a bud vase for small flowers and the second quite a bit larger with a wider neck to accommodate bigger arrangements. This gave me some flexibility on what to bring. Every other week I'd purchase one or two larger bouquets, and over the course of the week, I would pull out those flowers that had wilted and make a new creation in the smaller vessel with any stems worth saving.

I entered through the front doors one day with two bouquets that I cradled in my arm like an infant. I rounded the corner and a woman exclaimed, "Oh, boy, someone's getting flowers!" I looked at her and she was walking with her left elbow interlocked with...my mother! Mom recognized me and I discovered that the lady wasn't another resident rather a friend that was visiting the area from Florida.

Mary was one of the girls from Mom's time working at the hospital after high school. She had stopped by the house to visit Mom a couple of years before and they had exchanged Christmas cards for decades. I'd been sending Mom's holiday cards for her from the time I arrived back in New York. I would do all the addressing and include notes then wait for a day that she was doing well and had her sign her name. I questioned how long to do this. I wanted the friendships to endure with those that had kept in contact over the years and taken the time to remember her. At some point I knew I'd have to write with bad news and it seemed weird for me to leave any gap in communication.

When I asked how she knew Mother Dear was there, she told me that Mom's brother told her when they saw each other at the local senior citizens' center. He hadn't been in communication with his sister in at least two years. No impromptu stops at the house, no cards, no nothing. I could understand that he "just didn't want to see her that way." It's a common feeling we all have when confronted with a declining loved one. While I was willing to cut him some slack, I'm sure it was more difficult for my brother and me to see it happening to our mother than it would be for him with his sister. It's painful for everyone but that pain pales in comparison to the person with the illness. Join the club. Suck it up and visit because it's the right thing to do. I considered avoidance as the ultimate in selfishness. People live with these diseases 24/7/365 and to give up an hour of your precious life while enduring some discomfort is the least anyone can do.

That day, Mary had brought Mom a mini rose bush that stood about 6" tall. She told me they'd been sitting outside in the courtyard and she was just returning Mom to the activities room. She'd found her there when she arrived. I led them both back to Mom's room, we chatted a bit, I placed the rose in the sunlight prominently next to the other plants, and then Mary was on her way.

* * *

On Mother Dear's 80th birthday, I brought a card, two bouquets of flowers, a little palm plant, some jelly candy orange slices, and a big box of Russell Stover chocolates. She was in a great mood, recognized me immediately, and gave me a big kiss. When I left, I was feeling very good and I think she was, too!

I learned that when it came to celebrations, it was best to forego bringing anything of sentimental value since the concept would be lost on her. She didn't understand cards, and once placed in her room, were never acknowledged again. They were barely acknowledged when initially presented to her.

I brought fresh flowers every week until I realized that she didn't spend much time in her room. Aside from sleeping, she was never in there. For the most part, she didn't even know she had a room. The flowers would sit by themselves in a darkened room waiting for adoration that never came.

A year later, when I arrived on her 81st birthday, the staff was smiling and quick to point out that it was Mom's birthday. They said she'd had a great day so far. Unfortunately, she didn't recognize me and couldn't follow my explanation that it was her birthday. When I told her she was 81, she stared blankly as her brain failed to process the information.

We had a pleasant surprise that afternoon — her brother came to visit. He had stayed away because it bothered him to see her level of dementia and it reminded him of what might become of him. It was a shame he couldn't get beyond it because the main reason that particular facility was chosen was due to its location five minutes from his house.

He was three years younger and had all his wits about him. He took after his mother (my grandmother) who was mentally aware up until the time she died. It was my grandfather that had dementia and my mother had taken after him.

In addition to a card, he brought a newspaper clipping of an article from 1938 that recognized each of them for perfect school attendance. A photo of them both standing outside their home accompanied the news item. I suppose it helped your attendance when your mother was the teacher in a one-room schoolhouse!

Mom didn't recognize either of them in the picture and didn't know who he was as he sat beside her. She would have been thrilled to see him if she had understood. There had been times when she would cry and wish for him to visit when she was still at home with me. She was hurt and disappointed. That was in her mid-stages of dementia when she would have known him but immediately forgotten that he'd visited once he left. It really was a shame that her only sibling didn't visit more when she could have recognized him.

For where she was at in life — location and the disease — her birthday turned out to be a pretty good day.

* * *

Words you never want to hear your mother's nurse say: "There's been an incident."

She read a report describing how Mom had slapped two attendants and tried to bite a third when they were trying to get her to go to bed. The doctor on call was contacted and he prescribed a drug to calm her down. I expressed some alarm but it never happened again.

The nurse felt it was probably the attendants' approach and that the facility had recently been holding training classes on the subject of dealing with people suffering from dementia. I figured if they were close enough to get slapped, they must have been trying to physically force her. From my Mom's perspective, she was alone in an unfamiliar place and strangers were trying to force her to do something she didn't want to do. Like cornering a frightened animal, if she felt threatened, she was going to react.

I offered my opinion that if she didn't want to go to bed, they should wait five minutes and ask her again because she was likely to be in a completely different frame of mind.

Poor Mother Dear. Those were the things that broke my heart. They're the experiences that reinforced the correctness of our decision to place her in assisted care. It was better for her, and for us, that she had a team of professionals to manage her care instead of going through this alone at home.

CAST OF CHARACTERS — THE MEN

All of my life I've come up with nicknames for people — mostly for those who I don't know their real names. I have a rich fantasy life where I imagine what lives are being led by the people that surround me. Their clothing can draw my attention, or their mannerisms, ethnicity, body shape, daily schedule, or other completely irrelevant and random fact that happens to stand out.

For instance, the woman that used to leave our apartment complex in California at 4 a.m. became known as The Donut Lady because I imagined she must have been going to a donut shop at such an early hour. During the 1980's, there was a television commercial for Dunkin' Donuts depicting a man who was obsessed with getting up early to make the donuts. I figured this must have been the life of the The Donut Lady who needed to make sure the shop was stocked with freshly made glazed and powdered sugar breakfast treats in time for the morning rush. I found out later that she was getting up to work out at the gym. She was a stay at home mother and her alone time began before her husband left for work. She stayed home with the children for the remainder of the day. Never mind all that. She was still The Donut Lady to me.

Then there was the local attorney that talked directly into the camera in his television ads, assuring the viewer how he had their best interest at heart and that he'd fight and win on their behalf. Unfortunately, he showed a striking resemblance to a certain rodent despite being draped in a well-tailored suit with broad shoulders. He was known as The Woodchuck.

The tall, strapping man with incredible flexibility who practiced his martial arts skills by sparring with his reflection in the sliding glass door of his apartment became The Karate Kid. He would stand perpendicular to the window, bend sideways at the waist to the left and raise his straight right leg over his head, then simulate kicking someone in the face. Clearly, he was a teacher and not a student. These exercises went way beyond "wax on, wax off."

There was the elderly Vietnamese woman who lived with her extended family. She shared the apartment with one of her children and their spouse, and two grandchildren. Every afternoon she'd walk a lap around her apartment building for exercise and fill her lungs with the fresh ocean breeze of the Pacific, shuffling along the sidewalk in a gauze ankle length dress. Her face was very wrinkled, silently expressing years of experiences unknown, reminding me of an old-fashioned craft doll with a dried apple used for its head. She was known as Grandma Vietnam.

Lastly, there was the single mother living below with her daughter and sister. The sister liked to "entertain" men who climbed in and out of her bedroom window at all hours of the night. But she isn't going to be the subject described here. The mother was a Roseanne Barr-ish creature: short, heavyset, rotten disposition, and a loud mouth to match. If you were the casting agent looking for a female wrestler to be featured in a gritty made-for-TV movie, you'd need look no further. Taking a cue from the stage name of a professional male wrestler popular during the 1960's, my downstairs neighbor morphed into Mamma Bull Ramos.

With this sampling, it should come as no surprise that I had encountered a richness of characters practically begging to be nicknamed at my mother's assisted care facility.

Houdini

Houdini, the escape artist known for his propensity to leave the building unattended, came down the hallway and stood along the wall across from where Mother Dear and I were seated. When he was sundowning, he went from one exit door to the next to get outside, triggering the alarms each time.

He stood there for a while, looking back and forth at each of us, then crossed the hall and stood beside me. Being watched makes me uncomfortable; he had one bad eye and could barely see out of the other.

I considered that he wanted my seat, so I told Mom I was going to her room to check on things. I went down the corridor and made sure everything was in order. I watered the plants, which were doing surprisingly well. The furniture had been rearranged and it looked like they'd come through and steam cleaned the carpet.

When I got back, Houdini was sitting where I had been. I guess I'd become pretty in tune with these folks and determining what they wanted by their actions. It was dinnertime, and an attendant came down to take him to the dining room. His dinnertime was the same as my Mom's so she decided to guide her to the dining room as well and save a trip. Houdini stood up, took my Mom's hand to help her up, and away the three of them went down the hall to supper holding hands. I thought of Dorothy, the Scarecrow and the Tin Man. "Follow the yellow brick road. Follow the yellow brick road. Follow, follow, follow, follow, follow the yellow brick road." They did everything but skip!

Houdini could also be abusive. He was like Forrest Gump's box of chocolates — you never knew what you were gonna get. I always smiled and said "Hello" to make sure I stayed on his good side. He approached my brother one day and extended his hand to shake. As they clasped right hands, Houdini took a tight grip and pulled back his left hand in a motion to indicate a punch was the next item on his mind's agenda. After some quick talking, my brother was able to assure him that they were friends and he dropped his stance and smiled.

The Jackrabbit
Having the place a bit warm worked to Mom's advantage. Her room was on the north side of the building where opening the windows provided enough ventilation to keep things comfortable.

The activities room was where most of the residents spent their days. Aside from being the location for almost all of the daytime action, it was the only part of the building with air conditioning, the place where everyone congregated to keep cool during the hot and humid summer months.

There were plenty of tables where the Activities Directors coordinated games of bingo or conducted other inclusive activities. There was a fancy upright piano, donated by a neighbor, standing in the corner. Love seats and chairs were aligned to face a large screen television mounted on the wall. It was always tuned to the *TV Land* cable channel because the programming appealed to this age group. Oldies like *Bonanza, Gunsmoke,* and *The Andy Griffith Show* were on during the afternoon. Considering the age of the residents, the reruns on *TV Land* were from the years that these elderly folks were watching them in first run during prime time.

Each of the residents' rooms was equipped with a cable television hookup so those interested in keeping to themselves or watching something else could always retire to their rooms and enjoy a different show.

The Jackrabbit had his specific place in the recreation room. He sat, day in and day out, in the same chair at the back of the room. He rarely spoke, a combination of being shy and feeling self conscious about a speech impediment.

A man went into the bathroom located in the back of the activities room next to The Jackrabbit. He left the door open and everyone had the distinct pleasure of listening to him tinkle. The man was no sooner out of the bathroom than The Jackrabbit leaped from his chair and ran in. At first I thought the sound might have reminded him that he had to go as well. Instead, I saw him pull a length of toilet tissue from the dispenser, wipe off the seat, and give the commode a flush.

Most of the elderly men had poor aim and went all over the place. The bathrooms that were accessible to everyone were no exception. Their eyesight was compromised to begin with so imagine the additional challenge presented to an octogenarian with dementia. It must be frustrating to work in this type of facility knowing that as soon as you clean up a mess, the next person was going to immediately foul it up all over again.

About a half hour after I watched this performance of the bathroom shuffle, a woman went to open the folding doors where the games and activity items were kept. The Jackrabbit sprung into action, carefully pushing the doors closed and using his hands to indicate that she wasn't allowed access to the cabinets. She understood, took her walker, and went on about her business.

It was pretty clear that The Jackrabbit knew quite a bit about what was going on and kept an eye on the others. He made sure his corner of the recreation room operated in an orderly, clean, and safe fashion.

It wasn't too long before a female resident sat beside him and tried to engage him with the teddy bear she held on her lap instead of her usual doll. She "babbledy babbled" at the little brown stuffed animal with large yellow faux-glass eyes and appeared to be explaining what the bear was thinking. The bear was carefully given an imaginary drink from an empty plastic cup. She warned the furry little one that it was going to have to make a trip to the restroom if it kept drinking so much water.

The Jackrabbit watched her with his peripheral vision and

consciously chose to ignore her. He continued to sit as he did every day, staring forward and barely making a peep — until he needed to tend to something urgent that happened in his part of the world. When she reached for his arm to get his attention and explain her bear's current dilemma, he gently pushed her hand away but never made eye contact. I wondered how long this dance between the two had gone on? Did this only happen that particular time or was it a constant struggle that had been going on for years? Was it like a science fiction plotline where two conflicting entities are trapped in close proximity and destined to struggle for eternity?

The Jackrabbit permanently gave up his seat and began to stay in his room after Houdini physically threatened him.

The Preacher Man
A great life spirit and witty sense of humor is what you noticed first about The Preacher Man, a former minister. Round around the middle, with squinty eyes, a button nose, and fringe of white hair that framed his bald noggin. He was an endearing fellow.

A birthday celebration was in full swing when The Preacher Man entered the activities room. He burst into a boisterous rendition of *Happy Birthday* and led the entire room in song as he waved his imaginary conductor's wand to keep us all on the beat. As quickly as he appeared and struck up the band, he disappeared down the hall out of sight.

Pittsburgh
Pittsburgh was one of the first residents I thought was going to be a friend to Mother Dear. He liked the swings in the courtyard and would be sitting with Mom during her first weeks there. The staff told me that he'd declared that my mother was his girlfriend.

He was a loner that stayed in his room most of the time to watch television and sat by himself at dinner. Handsome, a short moustache, and almost completely bald. He didn't speak much, either, unless he became angry. When confrontational, I saw him put up his dukes and brush the sides of his nose with his thumbs like he was Rocky in a boxing ring.

Because he wore clothing that showed his support for NFL football's Steelers, I referred to him as Pittsburgh.

The Wolf
The Wolf was similar in demeanor and kept mainly to himself. He

was tall, slender, salt and pepper mustache, tattoos on his forearms, and a full head of hair cropped closely on the sides that stood straight up on top. His outfit of choice was a baseball cap, a jacket covered with sewn-on patches illustrating his many years in the Navy, blue jeans, and cowboy boots. If I had to guess based on stereotypes, I'd say he was a Texan.

The female residents referred to him as The Wolf because he kissed the ladies. His affections weren't focused. He was willing to get close to any woman that didn't rebuff him.

He was also the star of the "daring diaper caper." Standing in the corridor outside his room, stark naked except for his diaper, he tried to coax female passers-by into his room for fun and frolic. Not one of his finer moments, I'm sure.

Men, with their personalities, quirks, and natural tendencies presented a unique challenge.

SEXAGENARIANS

If there was any doubt that there was a potential for sex within the confines of an assisted living facility, witnessing the antics of The Wolf with his paramours was a real eye opener.

Call me naïve, but I just hadn't thought much about it. Yes, there were the jokes and stories about erectile dysfunction drugs changing the relationship landscape in nursing homes. They brought mental images of horny old men chasing the women, their crippled hands rolling themselves along in their wheelchairs, tongues hanging out, and arthritic fingers pinching all the butts that walked nearby.

But Mom? No way. She was in her early 80's so that shouldn't be any concern. My mother was practically a virgin, for God's sake!

My blissful ignorance came to a screeching halt when I walked in on The Wolf and Mother Dear engaged in a passionate embrace and kissing in the activities room. Activities indeed!

I was flabbergasted, and my jaw just about hit the floor in utter shock. I surprised them when I cleared my throat and asked, "What's going on here?" The Wolf jumped up and left without a word and I sat down next to Mom who seemed oblivious to what had transpired.

I had to let the scene sink in before I decided what to do. First, I couldn't chastise Mom because she didn't know what she was doing even if she "knew what she was doing." I couldn't really say anything to The Wolf because I was a visitor and had no right to discipline him. He wouldn't have understood or remembered at his level of dementia anyway.

The best option for me was to keep perspective and alert the staff of the shenanigans. When I told the nurse in charge of my Mom's care, she wasn't the least bit surprised. This had been going on for some time and since my Mother wasn't rejecting or resisting him, she said there wasn't a whole lot they could do.

Au contraire, mon frère!

I stewed on it for the next couple of days. I examined my personal reaction. Was I jealous that Mom liked someone? Did I think she was disrespecting the memory of my father? Could I be standing in the way of her happiness?

I had encouraged my mother to get more socially active in community activities to make friends and potentially find a special man after my father had died. A contractor that performed some carpentry repairs on her house had asked her to lunch. She declined, but I was very supportive and told her that it would be okay to go on dates.

That was before she started showing signs of mental illness. Mom hadn't been in a frame of mind to make any decisions about herself and her life for some time. She wasn't able to say "no," or "yes" for that matter, to ordinary life circumstances and decisions let alone physical contact or a sexual advance.

If a person isn't able to give consent, yet someone takes advantage of them because the person can't reliably resist verbally or physically, what is that called? Molestation? Rape? If a person with dementia consents, is it really consensual? What if the person making the advances has dementia? How would that be any different than a staff member committing the act? It's a very gray area.

I discussed the incident with my brother who didn't seem as alarmed as me. Regardless, I still knew I needed to do something. Once I sorted out that my initial reaction had been proper and measured considering what had happened, I evaluated next steps.

Reporting the situation to the administration was a great way to go because they needed to be aware of what was going on and I could seek their counsel. I was sure this hadn't been the first time they had dealt with this. I came to believe that they had seen it all.

I stopped by their office and asked if I could speak with them about something important. When I raised the topic, I found out that the nurse who I had originally talked with had reported my concerns. To their credit, the administrators had already taken steps to prevent a recurrence. The entire staff was made to sign a notice that described the situation and that interaction between my Mom and The Wolf was to be monitored and curtailed. Efforts were to be made to keep them apart as a preventative measure. The proactive stance and understanding put me at ease.

My role in Mom's life had become that of protector. It was up to me to ensure that she was safe since she had become so vulnerable.

And so it was. An unexpected hurdle overcome.

Retired U.S. Supreme Court Justice Sandra Day O'Connor had gone through something similar with her husband. Although there were no lurid details, it was reported that her husband had fallen in love with someone else that resided in his facility for people with Alzheimer's. It was described as a romance and that Justice O'Connor felt a sense of relief because he was happy after going through a painful time.

Experts say that it is somewhat common for Alzheimer's patients who forget their spouses to develop affectionate feelings for someone else. Even though patients lose their cognitive abilities, it seems the need for interpersonal contact and relationships doesn't go away.

CAST OF CHARACTERS — THE WOMEN

Not to be outdone by the men, the women provided a whole host of traits that were humorously noteworthy.

The Klepto
In any place where folks live communally with access to each other's rooms and the plentiful items found within, there's bound to be cases of sticky fingers walking away with things that are not one's own. Mix in the fact that the majority of the people don't know where their room is, let alone what is or isn't theirs, and you've got the ideal setting for musical chairs with personal objects.

I discovered that the disappearance of items was a routine occurrence. It's the nature of the beast. All clothes, including shoes, were marked with the resident's name using permanent magic marker. If a garment went missing, it would eventually show up in the laundry and be routed back to its rightful owner's closet.

When I refer to one of the residents as The Klepto, it is without judgment. She didn't know any better. These folks wandered in and out of rooms with no sense of personal space, property, or propriety and were liable to pick up something that struck their fancy and took it with them. They're like crows. They spot something shiny and interesting, stare at it, then nab it and take it back to their nest.

Some residents, however, exhibited this trait more than others. And so it was with The Klepto. When something was missing, the staff went to her room first because it was a fair gamble that the item had made its way back to her place. A bevy of looted treasure lied therein.

After Mother Dear's first couple of weeks, the nurses told us that Mom wasn't eating. A friend recommended that I bring her fattening treats so I delivered cookies, chocolates, and other sweets. Part of that stash was candy orange slices coated in sugar.

At home, Mom couldn't walk past the dish that held them without helping herself. They were kept in a covered plastic container and she didn't have any trouble identifying them, prying off the lid, helping herself, and replacing the lid to maintain their freshness. Before I purchased anything, I had to consider whether she'd know what they were and how to access them.

I set everything up on Mom's nightstand. About a week later, my brother was visiting in her room. Mother Dear was relaxing in the chair; he was lying across the end of the bed. In walked The Klepto. She marched past my brother, looked him in the eye as she passed, continued on to the end table where the goodies were kept, pulled open the drawer, and picked out two orange jellies. She looked back at my brother, popped them in her mouth, then turned around and left. Not a word was spoken by anyone.

It was all very innocent. I reported the event to the staff because I was worried that the high level of sugar content could pose a health risk if she was diabetic. Happily, she wasn't on a restricted diet and there was no cause for alarm.

Now, if I didn't know her as The Klepto, I probably would have nicknamed her Kentucky Derby. In the finest tradition of that event, she paraded around the place in bright floral-patterned dresses with huge hats that cascaded with silk flowers. Perfect for a day at the races!

Smoochie

Smoochie appeared to be one of Mother Dear's best friends at the place. They were usually sharing a swing and enjoying the wonderful summer weather in the courtyard when I arrived. Smoochie aggressively pursued sexual contact. In other words, she was the resident tart and The Wolf was her main squeeze.

On one particular visit, fully a year before The Wolf and Mother Dear became an item, I was talking to the staff in the lobby while watching Mom and Smoochie on their swing. The Wolf went out into the courtyard and sat on an adjacent swing. A minute later, Smoochie got up and hurried over to join him. Within seconds, they were attached at the mouth and going for broke. It looked like they were using their tongues to perform mutual tonsillectomies. Their ability to hold their breath, or breathe whilst making out, was a feat to behold as their lips were locked for what seemed like an eternity.

A member of the staff confirmed that she had two regular

gentlemen callers — The Wolf and Pittsburgh — that were the objects of her affection. Whether they made it to home base isn't of any interest to me since first base was all I was willing to observe or consider in my mind's eye. Their sexual behavior was hard to control and they couldn't be taught that physical expression was best saved for behind closed doors.

There were times when Mom thought that Smoochie was a man. She flirted with her, coyly waving as she passed and made room for her to share a swing. When reminded that Smoochie was a woman, Mom would blush, laugh, and think I was trying to fool her. Other times, she referred to Smoochie with female pronouns so it was hard to tell what Mom was thinking.

In fairness, I can't place complete responsibility for the lewdness on Smoochie since we already know that both of these men were ready, willing, and able. It takes two to tango. Or, in this case, three to tango, two at a time.

The Baby Mama

Roaming the halls clutching a doll at all times was The Baby Mama. She was very attached to the baby that she held so dear. The staff knew that if anyone wanted to cause a major ruckus, they simply needed to take it away from her. Boom, World War III!

The affection for dolls and/or stuffed animals is a common occurrence among the elderly. It could be that they need something to soothe their fears about unfamiliar surroundings, occupy their time, and fulfill a need to nurture something, or use it as a surrogate in place of their missing children. I suspected that for many of them, these inanimate objects were the only way they could express and 'receive' affection. The Klepto walked around with a large teddy bear most of the day. Another cradled a stuffed gingerbread man — a Christmas-time gift from her daughter.

For the most part, The Baby Mama was pretty incoherent when it came to language. A common condition as the brain deteriorates. Often the person knows what they want to say but they can't get their vocal chords and mouth to say it, causing a fair amount of frustration. A bit like being in a foreign country where you don't know the language. You know what you want to say; you just can't say it in the way that others can understand. Or maybe it's like a fussy baby. The baby knows what it needs but can only communicate through crying and gibberish.

The Baby Mama talked like a toddler, "Bah bah bah bah..." with a few words thrown in that were vaguely recognizable. Usually they didn't seem related to anything that was going on at the time where context clues would assist with their meaning.

Mother Dear and I were sitting and The Baby Mama walked by:

Me: Oh, look. She's got a baby!

Mom: That's not a real baby, you know. She's crazy.

There it was. Mom could identify a doll versus a baby and knew the status of the people around her. I realized, even if she didn't, that she herself might be clutching something meaningful somewhere down the road and have others consider many of her actions crazy.

Socks

Socks was forever shoeless. I'm sure she had shoes but preferred not to wear them. She enjoyed the courtyard, choosing to sit in a stationary chair in the shade rather than taking a place on the swings. I spent a lot of time on the swing with Mother Dear when I visited so I saw Socks all the time. We smiled, nodded, and said 'hello' to each other. The bottoms of her white sweat socks had become gray from the dirt and bits of leaves picked up from the cement patio. Truth be told, I'm a 'socks' myself when it comes to being around the house. I have always hated wearing shoes and usually walk in my stocking feet or barefoot down the driveway to retrieve letters from the mailbox or the newspaper from the sidewalk. I've learned to compensate by using a lot of bleach in the wash. Maybe I'm closer to assisted living than I think!

I'd estimate that Socks was about two years behind my mother in terms of her ability to remember. She struck up a long conversation with me in her southern drawl and she remembered everything about her past including the current status of her son, daughter-in-law, and grandchildren. She talked about her taxes and how selling her house impacted her income tax deductions. She missed having the property but not all the work required for the upkeep.

Yet, she asked me five times in the span of 20 minutes if I was my mother's only son. Each time I answered a different way to see if I could get the information to stick with her. But it didn't. Her immediate short-term memory was shot and that really is the beginning of the downhill slide.

She told me about her son's job, and how her grandchildren were in college while working and getting scholarships to pay for it. She had moved from South Carolina and had lived there at the facility for six months. On a separate visit, she told my brother that she'd only been there for three weeks. I inquired with the staff and found the truth was that she'd been living there for almost two years!

I felt sorry for her, my Mom, and all the residents when Socks told me, "This is a really lonely place."

Twinkle Toes

Twinkle Toes was a bit of a misnomer. Her eyes twinkled, not her toes, but for some reason Twinkle Toes seemed to fit and 'toes' is always paired with 'twinkle' in my mind. She had very bad curvature of the spine and walked hunched over. She reminded me of my Grandma whose spine had curled into the shape of a question mark, forcing her to face down towards the ground while standing.

Twinkle Toes seemed to be on a constant quest for something. She paced the halls with her painful-looking posture. Compared to the time when I first started visiting Mom, there seemed to be fewer people and the place seemed so much smaller. The faces were more familiar and the building's layout wasn't an unexplored mystery anymore.

I found Mom in the activities room shortly after I arrived. She was watching them play Wii bowling on the big screen television. Each of the players had a 'Mii' avatar and the facilitator was animatedly carrying on to make it interesting for the whole room rather than just the three that were able to play. In the meantime, he kept telling Smoochie to keep her hands to herself since she was canoodling with one of the men on a sofa.

I joined in with cheers for the strikes and spares, 'oohs' and 'aahs' for the near misses, and groans for splits. I wanted Mom to be more invested in what was going on. She had been an avid bowler back in her day with a league average around 160. I think my vocal participation and encouragement helped motivate the bowling players as if they had a bit of a rooting section behind them.

When it was time to eat I walked about two paces ahead of Mom so she could follow my lead. She not only forgot where we were going but how to get there. Her attention span was nonexistent and everything along the way served as a distraction.

Twinkle Toes was giving her attendant a hard time ahead of us. I'd seen her do that before, abruptly pulling her arm away when one of the nurses tried to take her hand and guide her somewhere. A not-so-subtle nod to stubbornness coupled with an exercise of independence.

Then everything changed when she spotted me. Twinkle Toes was pointing at me and smiling with a glint in her eyes. I'd never heard her speak but I could tell she was indicating something to the attendant about me.

Attendant: [To Twinkle Toes.] Yes, he's bringing his mother in to dinner.

Twinkle Toes held up her hand to me as we approached, and I took hers in mine.

Attendant: [To me.] Do you know her?

Me: [To attendant.] No. [To Twinkle Toes.] But I sure do see her around all the time. We pass each other in the hall and I see her in the activities room. In fact, she sits right across the table from my Mom at dinner!

Twinkle Toes's smile grew wider and her cheeks plumped up, forcing her eyes into thin arcs. It reminded me of Santa Claus and how he's usually depicted in illustrations for *'Twas The Night Before Christmas*.

I let go of her hand.

Me: Okay, everybody, let's go. We have to sit down because it's dinnertime!

Twinkle Toes turned and headed right for her seat. What had been a struggle of persuasion a few minutes earlier with the aide became easy. That is an effective method of getting someone with dementia to do something. Oftentimes, they resist, exerting some control in a situation where they feel powerless. Changing the subject and approach can quickly improve the situation.

We walked to her assigned table and I sat Mom in her seat, pushed in her chair, and said my usual "Hello ladies" to the group already there. Those that used to be leery of my presence now smiled back. Those that could speak said "Hello" in return and sometimes I even got a "How are you?"

Twinkle Toes had never acknowledged me prior to this. The nurse told me that I resembled a nephew that visited her and she may have thought I was him. It gave me pause, and I wondered how far I should allow these relationships to develop.

Over time it had become obvious that Twinkle Toes liked me.

But, she didn't like my brother, sneering at him and imitating his laugh with a wild cackle of her own. She was silent, and we thought she wasn't capable of talking, until one of the other residents rubbed her the wrong way. Sternly warning, while she shook her clenched fist, "Get away from me, you bitch, or I'll knock you up side the head!"

Tiny
I know that this nickname is politically incorrect. You see, Tiny was a little person who stood about four feet tall.

She was in her mid 80's and a pleasant sort, quick to giggle, hummed tunes to herself, and liked to hear herself talk. She began to daydream aloud after finishing a game of Bingo, looking out the window and commenting to all within earshot that it was such a beautiful day.

A woman in a wheelchair seated next to her paid Tiny a compliment on her shoes. Holy crap, that was all it took. It was too late because the floodgates had been opened and I listened to 15 minutes of everything I ever wanted to know about those shoes.

"I found them in my closet. I didn't know where they came from. My daughter asked if I found them. I have two pair — these brown ones and a pair of black ones. I have to have them specially made because I wear a size two and a half D."

She went on and on, over and over. I bet the woman in the wheelchair wished she hadn't said a word. I sure did!

The Bitch
I shouldn't call anyone a 'bitch' let alone someone in this situation, but you'll see why in a bit.

The Bitch was confined to a recliner on wheels because she wasn't steady on her feet. As I sat with Mom in wooden chairs pushed up against the wall along one side of the lobby, The Bitch had been placed in her chair directly in my line of sight. She was on the opposite side along the windows that looked out onto the courtyard. There were about six residents in chairs and the nurses' station was to my left where there was a lot of activity of aides and attendants.

The Bitch started in, "I need help!" She repeated. And repeated. And repeated. Each time getting louder. The attendants pretty much ignored her because she'd been doing this all day. She didn't really need help but wanted unending attention.

I just kept my nose buried in my crossword puzzle and ignored her. Visitors were in a weird situation where you couldn't help anyone even if you really wanted and were able.

"I gotta go to the bathroom," she said as she upped the ante to get some attention. She repeated. And repeated. And repeated.

She took off one of her shoes and flung it towards me. "Can't any of you assholes hear me?"

No matter how many times you pay attention to someone with dementia, or how many times you explain that they aren't allowed to get out of their chair for their own good, they continue to do it. They aren't capable of understanding that they've been told the same thing for hours.

Unfortunately, it's a bit of crying wolf. The time when she really needed help, no one would be paying attention.

Perhaps she should have been in a nursing home where she could have more dedicated care instead of a place where residents were expected to be able to live with guidance but not constant monitoring.

At this point, the question was, does The Bitch deserve sympathy for her situation or scorn for her nastiness?

The picture became clearer.

Nurse: I gave her a piece of gum and she called me a tramp!

My brother had a run in with her that was similar to mine. The setup was the same. The Bitch was in her wheel chair by the windows and my brother was against the opposite wall, facing her, with my mother seated to his right.

The Bitch began to stare at him and he tried to ignore her glare that was burrowing into him. She used her feet to pull herself forward, finally facing him, with their knees about a foot apart.

The Bitch: [Loudly.] What are you doing here?

Brother: I'm visiting.

The Bitch: [Even louder.] You're an idiot!

I laughed when he told me the story. It reminded me of Betty Davis giving it to Joan Crawford in *Whatever Happened To Baby Jane?*

Rosemary, about five feet away, began to giggle. We had a great relationship with her.

Brother: Are you laughing at me?

The Bitch: Of course she's laughing at you. You're an idiot!

Rosemary: [To my brother.] You ain't seen nothing.

If she kept it up, it wouldn't be long before she would be asked to leave because the other residents, who didn't suffer from dementia, would get tired of the foul-mouthed dramatics. The room my mother occupied was made vacant by a man who had become abusive to other residents and he was given 30 days notice.

I caught sight of The Bitch's daughters when they visited. Daughter 1 was a big-boned woman, a farmer or trucker type, and looked like she could seriously kick my ass if I so much as looked at her sideways. I dubbed her Bruisilla. Daughter 2 looked like the American al-Qaeda sympathizer called Jihad Jane. Over time, I realized that my first impressions of them were too harsh and they weren't as scary as their appearances lead me to believe.

Within one family we had The Bitch, Bruisilla, and Jihad Jane running around the place.

I did find some sympathy within my cold feelings towards The Bitch. One day I found her whimpering and crying alone in her wheelchair in the hallway. I asked if there was anything I could do, get for her, or take her anywhere that would help. She said "No" but seemed to feel better that someone had acknowledged her and asked.

Pufnstuf

She seemed quite young; I'd say late 50's, with dark hair that was about 25% gray and cut in classic style.

During her acclimation period, she walked the halls and went in circles in the lobby. She kept saying that someone was going to bring her things to her. On the surface, that sounded about right, until I realized she didn't even know she was staying there. Expecting guests may have been part of her behavior before she arrived.

A girl came around with a stainless steel service cart to offer midday drinks. This helped keep the residents hydrated. When asked if she wanted a drink, Pufnstuf replied "No." But she did want drinks for three other people whose names she gave — perhaps her children? The server came up with a clever answer, replying that everyone was required to come and get his or her own drink.

She was given a little carton of milk with a straw and didn't know how to drink it. I noticed on Western-themed Day that she had been given a small root beer float with a spoon and didn't understand what it was or how to eat/drink it, using two of her fingers to fish out the ice cream.

As she settled in, she continuously made quick puffing sounds similar to blowing out a lit match. She still wandered around lost and I often found her in Mom's room asleep on the bed. When she stopped to chat, she made little sense, trying to convey that there were people after her and watching everyone. Given her mental state, it made some sense that she would view the staff as captors since they tell everyone what to do, prevent them from leaving, and keep the residents in line if they're doing something that may endanger them or someone else.

Picasso

Picasso came to the assisted care facility during the summer. She had been in a couple of places before where they said she stayed in bed and resisted all efforts to get her up and about. Here, she had improved greatly. The staff was able to get her up, dressed, and out amongst the other residents.

She had some oddities, and could be a real Dr. Jekyll and Mrs. Hyde. She liked to attach herself to other women in the place and I'd noticed this behavior between her and my Mom. Picasso would sit next to them, caress their arms, tenderly kiss them on the shoulder, etc. She told them about going home and asked if they'd come home with her. It didn't really matter since no one was going anywhere.

On the other hand, she could get agitated and was quick to swear. She liked the term "sons a bitches." One afternoon she thought, courtesy of her paranoia and dementia, that they'd forgotten her for lunch. (I checked and she'd eaten.) But she went on a rant about how those sons a bitches had forgotten her. She said, "I'll take care of them!"

You might have thought, why had I chosen the nickname Picasso rather than Dr. Jekyll and Mrs. Hyde? Well, kittens, I'm much more clever than that!

It turned out that, like Picasso, she liked to "paint" shitty pictures. Let's just say she had a fondness for her own fecal material as a medium for art and liked to be creative with it, much to the dismay of the cleaning crew.

The Bugaboo

One of the biggest challenges was making sure that everyone got along. Certainly, I had noticed that some residents just didn't like each other.

The Activities Directors knew who were friendly and made sure they wound up sitting together on the various couches. Mom and The Bugaboo got along well.

The Bugaboo suffered from dementia; she could get the gist of what was going on around her but didn't understand the full story. I'd guess she was in her mid 70's and slightly better at reasoning than Mother Dear.

Her most obvious physical feature was a pointed nose that was well suited to her personality because she liked to poke it into everyone's business. That's why I referred to her as The Bugaboo. It's her ears, however, that were the most functional. She had a keen sense of hearing, and if folks were talking about something across the room, she'd go right over to offer her assistance. Not in a bad way, she just wanted to help.

This behavior got her into plenty of trouble with some of the grouchy residents. With the close living arrangement, many of the residents were irritated rather quickly if their personal space was invaded. The Bugaboo had earned her fair share of "Get away from me" and "Go somewhere else" comments. It didn't seem to hurt her feelings or mend her ways. She just moved on to the next bit of misadventure.

The staff liked to have The Bugaboo fold laundry bags full of towels and washcloths to keep her occupied and out of trouble. I know this is an activity that most assisted living residences employ because it is a relatively easy task and provides a sense of accomplishment. I told her how well she was doing and it was a big job that she had undertaken. She smiled wide, responded with some gibberish, and reached into the bag to get another item to fold.

Theresa the Activities Director (AD) decided that it would be a good idea to get a tabletop ironing board and an old iron, sans electric cord, in order to extend the amount of time The Bugaboo spent doing the clothes. The longer she kept busy, the better for her and everyone else. And without an electric cord, there was no danger present.

After hearing them talk about it for a month, the day finally came when the setup arrived.

Theresa: C'mon, it's time to work on folding the clothes. Ya gotta earn your keep around here!

The Bugaboo: I don't like the way you're talking to me. Are you trying to show off?

Ha! I remember hearing the same thing from my mother when I was growing up and I had gotten a bit too big for my britches.

Theresa: They aren't my clothes. Mine are at home. These are your friends' clothes.

The Bugaboo wasn't deterred and started folding the clothes and placing them on the table. The AD brought out the iron and ironing board, set them up on the table, and asked her to iron the clothes before she folded them. There wasn't any initial questioning, and The Bugaboo set to work. Then the light bulb went on...

The Bugaboo: Where's the electric cord on this thing?

Theresa: Oh, that iron is battery operated. It doesn't need a cord.

Hmmm, I thought, that was pretty quick thinking! The Bugaboo was satisfied and went back to work. The light bulb went on again...

The Bugaboo: [Pointing to the remaining stub of the electric cord.] What's this thing for?

Theresa: That's the antenna. The iron uses it to get its charge from the batteries.

That seemed plausible to The Bugaboo and she went back to the task at hand. The light bulb flashed back on again...

The Bugaboo: How come this iron isn't hot?

Theresa: It's child proof! It's the latest technology so kids don't get burned!

Damn, this story was getting better and better! I started to laugh and had to cover my face with the newspaper so I didn't spoil it.

One of the high-school-aged young men that worked there came in pushing the drink cart. "Ginger ale, cola, or water," he asked over and over, like a flight attendant moving down the aisle of a plane. He was offering a couple of shortbread cookies, too.

As he worked his way down the opposite side of the room, The Bugaboo started to repeat her line of questioning regarding the iron. This time, Theresa spun the tale wider and deeper. She talked about all the scientists involved in the creation of these newfangled devices, the level of technology involved, how expensive they were, etc.

Snack boy continued on from one person to the next, but he was listening, and his interest was peaked about the news he was hearing about such a fantastic new iron. I saw him being drawn into the farce, and as he turned around to ask more about the iron, we began to laugh. He blushed. The AD had been so convincing he'd bought into the story hook, line, and sinker.

Theresa: You oughta know better than to believe anything you hear around here at The Bullshit Hotel!

Lady Godiva

It wouldn't be entirely fair to the residents mentioned up until now if I didn't give my mother a nickname as well.

First, I will always know her as Mother Dear. I decided to step back and observe her and come up with a name by pretending that I was someone else's guest. How do they see her when they come to visit?

In her later years, Mom became increasingly sensitive to noise. "What's that racket," she'd demand in a belligerent tone when people spoke with raised voices, the kitchen staff was clanging pots and pans when preparing dinner, or the parakeets were squawking in their cages.

One reason I selected her particular room was because there was a birdcage outside in the corridor. She had always loved pets and we had a canary over the years. The parakeets, sad to say, became an irritation to her rather than a pleasure.

We were seated in the lobby next to a cage with two birds that had been together for eight years. Timmy, the larger green bird, was picking on Mimi, a yellow bird that was quite a bit smaller than her cage mate. They caused quite a commotion when the weaker one decided she'd had enough of the bullying and began to fight back.

Mom grew increasingly annoyed and placed the tip of her pointer finger on the inside crease of her thumb's joint, gave it some pressure to load it with spring, and moved her hand toward the cage.

Me: What are you doing?

Mom: I'm going to flick that damn bird on the tail.

I convinced her that the birds were simply having a bad day and that flicking the bird, even on the tail, wasn't a very nice thing to do.

That spawned my first nickname for her — The Flicker. It didn't seem very catchy, and not very accurate on its depiction of the person Mom was, but it was a decent first pass.

That name was in place until I witnessed something much more fitting of my creativity and imagination, and Mom's personality and actions.

> "Lady Godiva was a freedom rider, she didn't care if the whole world looked..."

The only thing constant is change and the experiences of a day can quickly devolve from being really great to terrible.

I found Mom sitting in the lobby asleep in a chair. She was seated next to a card table that had been set up so the AD could clip, file, and paint some of the ladies' fingernails. I pulled up a chair and sat next to Mother Dear. She held the shoe and sock from her right foot in her hand. Not surprising because she'd been obsessed with how her shoelaces were tied. They were never quite right no matter how many times they were tied and re-tied.

When I placed my hand on her arm to let her know I was there, she jumped from being startled, and then stared at me blankly. She was in a really heightened state of confusion.

When she finally came around, she asked why I hadn't kissed her when I arrived. An odd request since I never kissed her hello or goodbye. My brother had just told me that she'd started doing something weird with him where she puckered up and asked for a kiss when she first spotted him. He wondered if she thought he was our father, or one of the other men in the place with whom she shared make out sessions. I wasn't so sure, thinking it was just something she'd started doing, or behavior she'd picked up from The Wolf or Pittsburg.

We sat for a while, chatting with the AD, various residents, and aides that passed by on their way to do more important chores. I was very social while there so everyone stopped to talk for a bit.

Mom looked at her shoe, mumbled something and started to get up. I questioned her on what she wanted and I was ignored. She had gone back into her own little world. She stood up and started to leave. The AD got up and offered her a cup of water and tried to persuade her back to the table to sit with me. No luck.

I watched as she shuffled down the hall towards the activities room. I felt like I didn't exist and to her I don't think I did. I thought this was the start of what it would be like when she didn't recognize me at all. She had been recognizing me as someone special that was nice to her. But she didn't know I was her son or related to her in any way. In fact, I don't think she comprehended the concept of family and people being related. She hadn't asked for her mother and father in a while and that was something she had been doing pretty consistently.

I waited for her to come back. In a few minutes, Rosemary told me she was asleep on a couch in the activities room. I went in and sat beside her. She was having a vivid dream — moving her feet, twitching, talking, and manipulating imaginary things with her hands.

Twenty minutes after that she woke up and started complaining about her sweater. She was pretty quick in getting the sweater pulled half way up over her head before I could stop her. I asked her what was wrong and I explained that removing her clothes wasn't acceptable. I commanded her to stop but she was oblivious to everyone and everything around her. It was like watching a train wreck in slow motion. You know it's going to happen but you're powerless to stop it.

I tried to restrain her arms and get the sweater back on. It was like trying to hold a cat that doesn't want to be held. They wriggle, squirm, and contort themselves until they get away.

Mom got the sweater off, with nothing on underneath except her birthday suit. She hadn't worn a bra in years, complaining that they were too constricting. I looked around the room, feeling half embarrassed and half helpless, to see the 25 other people in the room watching the whole performance.

I told her to place the sweater over her like a blanket. At least that covered her and kept her boobs from flopping around. I heard someone behind me say, "Oh, she does that all the time." Uh, oh.

As quickly as she had taken it off, she collapsed against the back of the couch, exasperated, complaining that she couldn't get her damn sweater *on*! I helped her pull it back over her head and that ended the burlesque show.

Then it was time for her to eat and for me to beat a hasty retreat. Lady Godiva was born!

I was mindful of acknowledging and speaking to the residents I came in contact with. I'd estimate that 75% of them did not receive visitors. Any recognition from someone may be the highlight of his or her day. What was easy for me to do could have meant the world to them.

DAILY LIVING

I had been advised that Mom was attempting to leave the building during the first couple of weeks she was there. It was somewhat expected since she had exhibited that behavior when living at home and had vowed to run away if she ever found herself restricted in such a place. Being confined where it was new and strange meant she was going to try to get home. Or at least someplace that she felt was where she belonged, even though her loss of memory meant there wasn't any place that would be familiar.

Besides the obvious safety issue, I was concerned that she might be considered a nuisance. I wasn't sure what behavior constituted acceptable and unacceptable. A man had been asked to leave because he had become belligerent and threatening to others and was removed from the community. Would causing a commotion by attempting to leave be a reason to ask my mother to leave? What was the threshold for misbehavior?

The more time I spent visiting, I came to understand that residents headed for the exits and tried to leave all the time. There were residents far worse than my mother. Houdini was known for heading straight for the external doors when given half a chance.

Trying to leave the premises was just one more thing that vexed the staff on a continual basis. It wasn't until I witnessed an 'escape' by Houdini for the first time that I saw how these things were handled.

Mother and I were in her room when the central alarm started to blare. Mom pressed her open palms against her ears to block out the noise. I wasn't quite sure what was going on until I saw two staff members sprinting down the hall past our door. Mom's room was about a third of the way down a wing with doors at the end that served as an emergency exit. Beyond the doors was a large green lawn, several acres in size, which was recently mowed. On nice days it extended an enticing invitation that was hard to pass up.

I leaped from my chair but by the time I got in a position to watch the ruckus, the aides were already out the exit doors and bringing Houdini back into the facility. The attendants were out of breath but he was unharmed and no worse for wear. As they approached, I stood with a smile. "He does that all the time," they reported with big grins.

Knowing that my mother wasn't the only one to do such things reinforced my sense of relief and it was comforting to see how quickly the staff was on top of the situation. All exits were alarmed with sensors that were wired to a master panel mounted on the wall behind the nurses' station reception desk. When the alarm went off, they looked to the centralized electronic controls to see where the breach had occurred.

Residents that were prone to wandering and didn't know where they were, like my mother, were fitted with a device on their wrist that looked a bit like a big watch. It was examined to make sure it was functioning every day during the afternoon check of the residents. The staff told the residents it was something to monitor their blood pressure — a keen idea. I realized early on that telling the truth wasn't necessarily that important. If you want someone with dementia to do what you needed him or her to do, a bit of trickery might be the most effective strategy. After all, they'll forget it immediately so the truth doesn't carry any real significance in their limited world. Never lying may be a great choice in leading one's personal life, and living by an "honesty is the best policy" mantra is a noble idea, but the truth can generate a ton of avoidable frustration in the world of Dementialand.

I'm not perfect.

I found Mom lounging sideways in a chair as she often did — a perpendicular position to the seat cushion with her back against one arm of the chair and her legs dangling over the other. Her chin was in her chest and she was sleeping.

The lobby chairs were popular and there was rarely a vacancy. A definite pecking order for prime seating existed. Some of the residents got up early to stake a claim on their favorite spot and remained there the entire day. Once someone left, someone else would get up and take the seat. Moving up to a better class of neighborhood, I suppose.

I squatted by her side, balancing on the balls of my feet, and spoke softly to her so she would know I was there. Her face lit up with recognition as her eyes opened and she wiped some drool from her chin. She sat upright and I tried to engage her in conversation.

When there was a need for extra seating, chairs could be retrieved from the chapel. I decided it was time to take a seat, as the arches of my feet grew weary. There had been a fire drill earlier in the day and most of the hall doors were still closed as they completed the testing of the alarm system.

I stood up, turned, and pushed through a door off the lobby. Immediately the siren sounded. I'd set off the alarm as if someone was leaving. I found myself looking at the outside of the building through the door I'd just opened, realizing I was the escaping culprit. I had mistaken a windowless outside door for the one leading to the chapel.

"It was me, it was me," I exclaimed. The residents were looking at me as well as the staff. "I thought this was the door to the chapel." I slunk sheepishly through the crowd and made my way around to the chapel. I waited a bit for the commotion to settle down before returning with the chair.

From then on it was hard for me to fault anyone for setting off the alarm considering I'd done it myself.

* * *

On a quick check of Mom's room, I noticed that the wastebasket by the window had quite a bit of urine in it.

I alerted the staff. What I thought was going to be a big deal barely made a blip on their radar because things like this were a common occurrence. They were in the room cleaning things up in two shakes of a lambs tail. People tinkled in their chairs, and by "their" I mean the chair they just so happen to be sitting in at the time — including the staff's desk chairs. Some residents peed in their pants, others peed in the plants. The fact that Mom actually hit a wastebasket and it was easy to clean up was a bonus. A cleaning lady told me that one resident had defecated in the sink of the common bathroom located off the lobby. She wasn't quite sure how he did it, but the evidence was impossible to miss!

I put on my detective hat and began to piece the puzzle together. Mother Dear must have awoken sometime during the night, had to go, didn't understand that she needed to locate a bathroom, and used the closest thing she could find. I gave her an "i" for ingenuity. She was aware that relieving herself in her pants wasn't correct and that these things needed be done into a container of some sort.

Since that happened, she had done 'number one' and 'number two' in the trash receptacle in her bathroom. It made no sense to a logical mind why she had done her business in a basket literally a mere foot away from the toilet. She must have been looking right at the toilet while she was going but made no connection between what she was doing and where it was appropriate. She had forgotten that toilets were for this activity.

A month later they pulled me aside and said that Mom was tinkling in her shoes. How does something like that happen? I figured that she must have been standing and that it ran down her leg into the shoe when she couldn't hold it anymore. No, they said, the shoes were full when they found them in her room. "Hmmmmm," I responded, "that's pretty good aim for a woman!" I hadn't considered that Mom had held the shoe up to herself before urinating until the nurse expressed how she thought things had gotten where they were.

Adult undergarments were used with her from then on to catch any accidents until they put her on a toileting schedule. She had the ability and knew enough to hold it. She didn't know enough to ask for help.

* * *

The path of her dementia yielded some surprises along the way. I had parked her bright red two-door Chevy Cavalier in the lot directly in front of the building. As she and I passed the front door on our way to the activities room, Mom spotted it, pointed, and commented about her little car. While she barely knew who anyone was, she remembered that car.

My brother stopped in to see her two days after that. She mentioned me by name and that I had just been there yesterday with her car. She told him she'd considered getting into the car to drive home but thought better of it. This demonstrated a great deal of awareness that she had about her situation.

The information was in her mind; it was just that the inhibited neural pathways caused by the disease that made it nearly impossible to access it. Sometimes the information managed to come forth but at a later time. She might respond to something that was said 15 minutes before. I don't know if her brain's circuits were slow or if they kept trying to find an alternate route to the data and eventually succeeded.

* * *

Two colors fell into the category of favorites. Mother Dear had a penchant for purple clothes and red nail polish. I brought red nail polish and some acetone remover to give her a manicure and pedicure. She enjoyed the physical human contact and felt special. When she was living at home, Marilyn had started field trips to a nail salon in a local strip mall as an adventurous way to get her out of the house for exercise and a change of scenery. Mom ended up with a crush on the young Vietnamese man who always tended to her so that made the outings even better.

I'm no nail technician but I did okay and she was happy. After allowing time for the polish to dry, I asked her if she'd like to go out and spend some time in the courtyard on one of the swings. She was quick to agree. We sat on a swing next to a woman who was in an adjacent swing, and three other residents were sitting in stationary chairs nearby.

Socks: [To me.] How long have you had that mustache?

Me: Oh, it's been years now.

Socks: Your nose is really big.

That'll be enough from the peanut gallery, thank you very much!

* * *

The lobby was a great place to sit for people watching. The staff came and went from the nurses' station, the courtyard was just beyond the floor to ceiling windows, the dining room was accessed through an entry in the corner, and all of the resident room's corridors converged there. The team from the activities department used the space, too.

So it came as no surprised when I arrived to find quite a spectacle. Plopped square in the middle of the lobby was a mat from the game Twister surrounded by a bunch of people in wheelchairs. I thought, "Now this is going to be interesting!"

Mother Dear was seated against the far wall so I grabbed a spare chair and took it over and sat next to her. She was about the same, sleeping sideways in the chair, and I pulled out my *USA Today* newspaper to do the crossword puzzle. Although I was sure there was going to be entertainment considerably more fulfilling occurring in front of me at any moment.

A portion of the lobby in front of the windows was kept clear of people, chairs, and sofas. I assumed this was due to fire code regulations. In came the bubbly AD Theresa, she of The Bugaboo's newfangled cordless iron ruse. I called over to her that I should have figured she was the one behind the hoopla.

The job of AD took a whole lot of patience and just as much ingeniousness. How do you keep 50 or more people entertained for eight hours a day? Then think about how the residents are in various levels of mental capability and an equally wide variety of physical capability. And a very tight budget. I gave them a ton of credit.

It turned out the game was "Pitching Pennies." The residents were allotted three pennies and the AD would go around the semi-circle of players and spin the dial. When it landed on a color, it was up to the resident to toss their pennies one at a time to see if they could get them to land on any of the correct color dots. It was something easy, entertaining, and they could all play at whatever level of health they were at. Theresa provided a lot of instruction, coaching, encouragement, assistance, and commentary throughout the game.

The whole scene grew as the game got under way. More residents arrived, stopping to watch out of curiosity. It turned out to be the most well attended game I'd seen take place over the entire span of time I had visited. This simple idea was easy to understand, execute, and proved very popular!

Playing on this winning theme, the game was modified at other times and applied to Bocce. It wasn't as popular with the residents (players or spectators) as Penny Pitching Twister had been but it was pretty well attended nonetheless. Perhaps the large plastic Twister mat was something that drew more attention.

In the Bocce game, the AD gently tossed a golf ball into the center of the play area. Each player was given two croquet balls of a color that were different from the others to roll towards the golf ball. The closest person would win that round. It was a bit like watching people at a bowling alley. Some rolled their balls smoothly, others tossed, and some just dropped them. Luckily the floor wasn't exactly level so those balls that were dropped wound up rolling, too.

I watched four residents participate, each with moderate dementia. One was in a wheelchair, one used a walker, and the remaining two were able to get around without assistance.

I noticed that the AD had made two teams of two, rather than each playing on their own, making sure there was twice the chance of winning. She would announce the closest as the winner and then include their teammate as winners of the round.

During the game, there was some mental stimulation.

Theresa: [To Resident 1.] You've got green balls. What things outside are green?

It was sad that Resident 1 looked directly outside at the courtyard but couldn't name anything that was green.

Theresa: [Helping.] Well there are the trees, the shrubs, and the flowers.

When it was another resident's turn:

Theresa: You've got yellow balls. What things outside are yellow?

Resident 2: The sun.

Theresa: Corrrrect! The sun is something outside that is yellow!

All the while, my mother sat in her chair and seemed oblivious to the activity occurring 10 feet in front of her.

I was more invested than she was, saying encouraging things like, "Oh, that one was close!" and "Great job!"

* * *

I had set aside four casual pairs of shoes and five sweaters to bring up for Mom. When I got to her place, I dropped them off at the office where they marked everything with her name. I continued on and joined her on the davenport where she was sitting. Her finger nail polish was chipping so I did her nails — stripping off the old enamel, clipping and filing them, then applying two coats of a new color. The other women (residents and staff) were a bit envious since they always joked about me doing theirs, too.

As the polish dried, one of the aides came down the hall. She was carrying the clothes I'd just brought, already marked with her name, to hang in my Mom's closet.

Me: [Excited.] Oh, look! All these new clothes are for you!

Aide: [Sits on couch next to mom, displaying items one at a time.] Look at all these new sweaters!

Me: I just did her nails. Pretty pink!

Mom held up her hands, wiggled her fingers, and grinned.

Aide: They're beautiful! I'm going to put all these nice things in your closet. They're all for you!

Mom: [Bottom lip quivering.] I'm really lucky.

At that moment, she thought she was. And my bottom lip was quivering as well.

* * *

Yet there were other days when she didn't feel quite so good about her situation.

The Baby Mama had peed her pants in the recreation room and she was soaked. An aide was trying to persuade her to go into the bathroom to change into clean clothes. She was a feisty old woman, though, and resisted all efforts. I'd seen her hit the aides in the chest with both hands — like Elaine on *Seinfeld* when she said her trademark "Get! Out!" — except Baby Mama said "No" and "Get away." She was making quite a scene.

Reinforcements came to help and two took a hold of each arm. They guided her to the bathroom with her complaining the whole way.

Mom: [Under her breath.] She's gonna get a beating.

I'm sure that wasn't the case, but as soon as someone says something like that, even if they have dementia, it makes you wonder.

* * *

After Mom complained about a sore that was developing on her upper lip, I talked with the nurse about a potential cold sore outbreak.

A woman, in the later stages of dementia, approached me. She was able to talk and form complete sentences. However, what she said wasn't rooted in reality. At least today's reality. She interrupted our conversation.

Woman: I can't find it.

Me: What are you looking for?

Woman: My car. Someone's taken my car and I can't leave.

Nurse: [Motioning with her arm.] Well this office is too small so your car isn't in here.

That was a bit of a mistake. While technically accurate, and seemingly enough information to get the woman to move along, it was providing a rational answer to someone who didn't understand rationality. To normal people, we'd deduce that the room was indeed too small to hold a car and move on. Not to someone with little or no reasoning skills. She stayed, looking concerned.

Me: What kind of car?

Woman: It's a Ford.

Me: [Pretending to jot down the information.] Okay, I'm making a note of it right now.

The nurse could see the tablet that I was holding and that I wasn't really writing anything.

Woman: It's blue.

Me: Okay, one blue Ford is missing. Got it. As soon as it turns up, I'll come and get you immediately!

It threw her a bit of a curve, bewildered that someone acknowledged her concerns.

Woman: Thank you. They've been taking a lot of people's cars. I didn't think they'd take mine, though.

Me: Oh, dear. That's definitely something we need to keep track of. I'll keep an eye out and maybe we can catch them.

The woman nodded affirmatively and pushed her walker down the hall. I turned back to the nurse to continue our conversation about lip balm for the cold sore.

Nurse: You need an application.

Me: What do you mean?

Nurse: To work here. You're really good with the residents.

It was an interesting observation. I guess I had a knack for going along with whatever I was being told. Contradicting them was pointless. I thought about elder care as a potential new career but I'd like to work in an office doing marketing rather than work the floor where I'd be constantly responsible for their health and well-being.

* * *

The things you see and hear can be hilarious or downright heart breaking.

———

The Bugaboo was walking through the lobby. She passed The Bitch who had her own sweater folded over the arm of her wheel chair.

The Bugaboo: [Reaching towards The Bitch's sweater.] Is that my sweater?

The Bitch: [Brushing The Bugaboo's hand away.] No. It's mine.

The Bugaboo shrugged and continued walking down the hall.

———

Aide 1 went to take Twinkle Toes to the bathroom. She resisted, causing Aide 1 to take her by the elbow to guide her.

Twinkle Toes: What're ya doin', ya damn fool!

———

Ten minutes later, The Bugaboo made another lap on her walk.

The Bugaboo: [Reaching towards The Bitch's sweater.] Is that my sweater?

The Bitch: [Brushing The Bugaboo's hand away.] No. It's mine!

The Bugaboo shrugged and continued on.

———

Aide 1 wheeled Tiny into the lobby and parked her wheel chair by the nurse's station.

Aide 1: [In a cheery voice.] There ya go!

Tiny: Rotten old bitch.

Ten minutes later, The Bugaboo headed towards The Bitch.

The Bugaboo: [Reaching towards The Bitch's sweater.] Is that my sweater?

The Bitch: [Brushing The Bugaboo's hand away.] No! It's mine! Now move along!

The Bugaboo: Well you don't have to be so nasty about it.

The Bugaboo shrugged and continued walking down the hall.

The Preacher Man was talking with Socks.

The Preacher Man: Sometimes I just want to go home and die.

Socks: I know. This place can get real lonely.

Ten minutes later, The Bugaboo made another lap as if it had been her first.

The Bugaboo: [Reaching towards The Bitch's sweater.] Is that my sweater?

The Bitch: [Brushing The Bugaboo's hand away.] No! It's mine! I've told you that before!

The Bugaboo: I know. Sheesh.

The Bugaboo wandered on. Part of me wondered if The Bugaboo knew exactly what she was doing and was trying to annoy The Bitch. I gave The Bitch credit for holding her temper as long as she did, given her rotten disposition, because I'd seen the exact same interaction between the two on many other days.

A new man was confused on his first day.

Resident: All I know is that they said we were going for a ride and I ended up here.

My heart felt so bad for him, and I had a pang of guilt because I'm sure that was how my mother must have reacted during her first few weeks. I asked the staff about it and they said he'd been there with his family to take a tour and had been told it was going to be his new home. Dementia — in one ear and out the other.

* * *

The head administrator of the facility brought in her little black Schnoodle (Schnauzer x Poodle) puppy. It was the cutest little thing you ever did see!

She brought it in to work a couple times a week and the residents were able to hold it on their laps, pet it, and cuddle it. It was amazing how everyone, including me, perked up when the dog was around.

Mother Dear missed her cats and saw their images in unlikely places. On many occasions, while I was sitting next to her, I'd have my legs crossed and rotate the free foot to stretch my ankle. Combine the motion with the fact that my sneakers were black and white, and Mom thought it was Pooh Pooh. She cooed and talked baby talk to my foot in a soothing voice.

Pet therapy is a good thing and I was happy the little pooch was around. It gave the residents a great substitute for the animals they'd left behind.

What I learned over time was that everyone had some sort of special issue, need, or personality quirk; otherwise they wouldn't be in an assisted care situation.

HOLIDAYS

The holidays can be a terrible time for those that are alone. If there's any saving grace about dementia, it's that those that suffer from it aren't completely aware of their condition. They aren't lonely on holidays because they don't understand what holidays are anymore.

Mom's first Thanksgiving away from home went very well. Their main meal was to be served at 11:30 a.m. and two guests were allowed per resident. I arrived shortly after 11 and found Mother Dear in the recreation room watching the Macy's Thanksgiving Day parade. Snoopy, inflated and tethered to his minders, was just making his way through Times Square.

Mom wasn't feeling very well and complained of a stomach ache. That was normally code for, "I have to go to the bathroom." Before we headed to the dining room, I took her to use the facilities in her room but that proved uneventful. A false alarm.

Seating began a few minutes later. I was placed at the head of Mom's table, to her left, and she sat in her regular seat. Two of her regular dinner mates had been picked up by their families and weren't there, leaving three others besides Mom and me. The room had been decorated with streamers, and turkeys with bodies made of honeycombed paper sat at the center of each table between placemats with a harvest design.

She was still holding her stomach when they served the meal. Mother started slowly but the other ladies said that she was a good eater and always finished her plate at every meal, eating more than each of them. She zoned out a couple of times and then came back from wherever her mind had gone and had to refocus on me and who I was. I gently suggested she just have some mashed potatoes and maybe that would calm her stomach. She ended up eating the entire meal once she got started.

They did an impressive job. Slices of real turkey (white and dark meat without bones), stuffing mixed with broccoli florets, mashed potatoes, butternut squash, cranberry jelly, and a roll. The plates were full with plenty of gravy poured over the meat and potatoes. Apple or pumpkin pie was offered as the final course. I chose apple and it seemed like they had baked it in the kitchen on premises. Mom requested ice cream, and the server returned through the swinging door of the kitchen with a scoop of vanilla with some chocolate syrup drizzled over the top. Enjoying every bit, Mom scraped the dish clean with her spoon. No wonder she had belly aches!

After she and I finished, I led her back to her room and turned on the television. I sat in the chair and watched the annual dog show while she lied on the bed, closed her eyes, and relaxed. I snuck out after she'd fallen asleep.

For twenty years, we watched the Macy's parade on television and then drove to visit my paternal grandmother who lived with my aunt and her family. I was always afraid of this grandmother even though she was nothing but sweet. I was ill at ease as a child because she never wore her dentures. She was about five foot tall, skinny, nice as can be, and always offered chocolates from a box with a map of the flavors printed on the inside of the top.

She was the youngest of nine in an Irish family. Hoosick Falls was filled with second-generation Irish and Polish immigrants in working-class neighborhoods. During WWII, she had been a sort of 'Rosie the Riveter' in a factory for the war effort. Her husband, my grandfather, had died in the 1940s, before my mother had met my father, remaining a mystery to his descendants. No one spoke much about him, and my grandmother remained a widow until she died in the late 1980s.

Finished with that visit, next was literally over the river and through the woods to my maternal grandparents' house we went. This grandmother was the most influential in my personal development and she was an incredible cook. Other than her culinary talents, where I have minimal interest, she is the person I have tried to model my life after.

My grandmother always put on a huge spread for Thanksgiving and dinnertime was promptly at 2 p.m. Everyone in the family had their favorite dish. As the years went by, poor Grandma worked like crazy to bring it all together for the group of us. She would be up at 4 a.m. to put the turkey in the oven, working in a small kitchen with a ceiling that drooped in the center and seemed on the verge of collapse.

There was the traditional turkey, with its perfectly browned breast, carved by Pop who always claimed the tail. The bird had been stuffed with dressing made with cubed stale bread, onions, celery, and Bell's seasoning. The potatoes were whipped with heavy cream and butter and accompanied by gravy of pan drippings that were thickened with cornstarch as my uncle liked it. Boiled onions were a favorite of my grandfather and the mashed turnip was the dish that Grandma prepared for herself. The baked oyster casserole was only really eaten by my mother and a few other adults who would dollop little scoops onto the edge of their plates. There was the annual dispute about what preparation of cranberries was the best — my father preferred jelly straight from the can whereas my aunt liked fresh berries chopped into a relish. The basket of garlic bread disappeared when it reached my cousin and the bowl of raspberry Jell-O with real whipped cream on top ended up parked in front of my brother. I was a fan of the banana bread, the location of the recipe still unknown, that reigned supreme when compared to any others I've eaten.

After a prayer, everything was passed to the right as it made its way to everyone seated around the heavy antique wood table. From my seat, I had a view of the curio cabinet with the collections of glassware and unique ceramic salt and pepper shakers.

There were freshly baked apple, mincemeat, pumpkin, and raspberry pies for those that had saved any room for dessert. The raspberries had been grown on the back of their property, picked during the summer, and frozen for just this purpose. Japanese beetle traps were placed among the rows to reduce the devastation their voracious appetite had on the raspberry canes, and grape leaves draped over an arbor. The hand-picked berries were tart but enough sugar was added to strike a perfect balance of sweetness. These pies were so delicious that we requested them in place of cake on our birthdays.

The men and children would retire back to the living room after the feast, unbutton the front of their pants, watch football, and "visit" (chat). Usually the men discussed deer hunting and the elusive eight-point buck they saw the other day. This was long before the local deer population exploded. It used to be that seeing a deer through binoculars was a rare sight; now they come up to the house's edge to munch on rose bushes and the foundation shrubs.

The women, bless their hearts, moved back to the kitchen to do the dishes and clean up. My grandmother didn't have a dishwasher so all dishes were done by hand. When they were finished, they joined the group for more talking. The conversation would usually change to discussions about relatives, neighbors, and friends with question like, "Have you seen so and so lately?" and "Do you remember when..." as they talked about old times. I know about a lot of people that I never met just from listening to the stories every holiday. This cultural art form, the passing of stories from one generation to the next, seems to have gone by the wayside.

Supper was at six where everything was brought out again, warmed up, and served as a buffet. The portions were decidedly smaller on this second grazing where a heavier emphasis was placed on the pies.

That was how we spent Thanksgiving every year when I was growing up. Turkey was served again at Christmas and ham at Easter. Green bean casserole seems to be a staple now but we never had it then. I look back on those times and can't believe my Grandma prepared such a huge, delicious spread well into her seventies!

* * *

While Thanksgiving was mainly just the special dinner at Mom's place and sparsely attended by the families, Christmas was a much bigger event at the old folks home. The common areas were decorated for the weeks surrounding the holiday season. The staff was divided into two sides for a team-building contest to determine which group could come up with the best theme. There were trees placed in every area large enough to accommodate one, replete with twinkling lights, tinsel, and featuring resident-crafted ornaments.

Again, each resident was allowed to invite two guests. The party wasn't held on Christmas day itself so more families attended. For this meal, the dining room was full and there were folding tables set up in the halls and lobby to accommodate everyone.

When my brother and I arrived, Mom was upstairs in the beauty parlor having her hair done so she looked great when we saw her. She recognized my brother but not me. He pointed directly at me and asked her, "Who's that?" She looked right through me. No clue. Her understanding of the world went up and down and I'd have rated that as a mediocre day for her.

The staff served shrimp cocktail as people arrived and mingled. Platters of cheese and crackers, crudités, and bowls of chips and pretzels were placed on the counters.

The call to dinner was at noon. They did a good job with the spread. Broiled lemon chicken breast (boneless, skinless), beef stroganoff, scalloped potatoes, stuffing, macaroni salad, mixed berry Jell-O, roll, and a strawberry shortcake layer cake for dessert. I overheard several people say that the food they had seen at other assisted living centers paled in comparison. Hearing those sorts of things reassured me that we made the right decision for Mom.

My brother and I compared notes about the experiences we'd had with the various other residents. We hadn't been there at the same time since the dropoff, having made the decision to each go up twice a week so Mother Dear had a visitor every other day. I went on Tuesday and Thursday, he on Friday and Sunday.

It was interesting to see so many of the children of the residents and how many looked just like their parents. Most of the folks that worked there confused me with my brother. It was easier to tell us apart when I had longer hair but that changed when I got a trim so we had similar haircuts. They never saw us together; a couple of people thought we were the same person. We do look alike. Like brothers, not twins, but whatever. The bad news for me was that they all thought I was the older brother but I'm nine years younger! I've chosen to think that my brother looks young for his age (he does) rather than I look old for mine (I hope not).

The staff had organized a program for the afternoon and the residents were all herded into the activities room. It began with a couple of singers that brought in a banjo to sing Christmas carols and most of the residents sang along. Songs are something that seem to withstand the ravages of Alzheimer's disease. Everyone chimed in to sing *Rudolph the Red-Nosed Reindeer* and *Frosty The Snowman*.

Halfway through the caroling, Santa showed up. A big man in a suit and I do mean BIG. He bellowed "Ho Ho Ho," shouted "Merry Christmas," and tried to pay special individual attention to each of the residents.

The AD had organized a gift exchange that was like a Secret Santa. All of the families received a note with their November invoice to buy a gift for a certain person that had been selected at random. An option, which we'd taken, was to give the staff $10 and have them purchase something. They knew the residents, what they needed and liked, and could make a better decision.

One of Santa's duties was to hand out the gifts. He'd call out the residents' names, they would raise their hands, and Santa delivered the present to them.

For everything that was going on, it all went off without a hitch!

I wanted to do something special and personal for the staff during the holidays. I had so many ideas. A $15 gift certificate so the ladies could get a manicure/pedicure to pamper themselves; the same for the men to get a haircut?

I spoke with the administrator who said that cookies or donuts in the break room would be appreciated and sufficient. That was what most of the families did that were interested in doing something. I didn't think that was personal enough. We tip our postal carriers, our paper delivery people, our hair dressers, our doormen — it just seemed right to tip the people who held my Mom's life and well being in their hands. Believe me, they earned every penny of their salary, and I think a little appreciation goes a long way.

There were 40 people to purchase for in total. This included the nurses, aides, administrators, activities department, and even the kitchen staff. I started to think of less expensive ways that would be nice but not perceived as cheap. What about a $5 gift certificate to the locally owned coffee shop for a latte and muffin? That would keep the money in the community by supporting a local business. After more consultation, I learned that many of the people that worked there didn't even have cars. Going to a coffee shop, even if it was down in the village about a mile away, wasn't such a good idea after all.

In the end, I opted for tins of Danish cookies. They were $2 each and had a special holiday design on the top. Some had a reindeer, some a snowman, and others had a poinsettia. I brought them in and the administrator said she'd be happy to distribute them for me when the workers came in to pick up their last check before Christmas. That was a relief because there were three shifts and I only knew those that worked in the afternoon.

On each, I affixed a tag. I wrote:

To: Thank You
From: Evelyn and Sons

Everyone received something individually as a show of thanks. It wasn't a lot, but it was something nonetheless. I know my Mom would have thought of something similar if she had been able.

Mother Dear always pulled out boxes and boxes of decorations for every holiday. The closets and attic held strings of lights, fancy ornaments, ropes of garland, and all manners of adornment cobbled together over the years. Christmas was a unique holiday in that the outside of the house was included in the trimmings. All of the evergreen shrubs were wrapped in lights with large multi-colored bulbs with blinkers interspersed, a large sign proclaiming "Noel" was placed above the garage door, electric-powered candles were placed in the front windows, and flocked wreaths were hung on the doors.

The Christmas tree took center stage in front of the picture window. Lights first, garland second, the ornaments, and then the icicles. Each of us had our own special ornament that we placed every year. My brother had the pink ball with a sparkling sun on the side and I had the white ball with a country scene painted on it. There were Santas, elves, sleds, and solid balls that functioned as filler. The icicles were delicately placed by hand with one strand individually draped on the tip of every branch. A silver and gold aluminum star with a yellow flashing bulb at its center was the topper.

One December night when Mom was still at home, I was a bit ashamed that our house was a dark blot on our otherwise brightly lit street. I had a twinge of guilt. I wasn't prepared to recreate the look from my childhood, but I wanted to do something, so I purchased three green and three red floodlights. That provided maximum effect with minimal effort on my part.

The effect of the lights reflecting against the white aluminum siding bathed the whole house in alternating green and red light. A striking view from the street. From inside the house, the lights glowed and illuminated the venetian blinds in the windows. Mom just couldn't figure it out. "What are all those damn lights?" "Who put those damn lights up?" "Someone's shining green lights in our windows and there's red ones in the bedroom." "I think the house is on fire." My explanation that they were holiday lights brought an understanding nod, until the next time she noticed them and said the same things.

The setup was a bit pricey at $100 for the bulbs, power strips, and extension cords, but any extra that I paid up front was more than made up for in the lack of labor to put them in place. No staple guns, tangled cords, or burned out bulbs. I realized an added benefit on the back end with the ease of taking things down. I just pulled up six stakes, wound up the cords, and that was that.

Why is it that every year it seems to take a lot more time to take things down than it ever did to put them up?

* * *

Yes, the activities team was inventive. I was always impressed with their creativity given that they operated on a shoestring. Hardly an opportunity went by for them to celebrate something. When you have 50+ people to keep entertained and engaged, you look for inspiration wherever you can.

What better way to keep so many happy and entertained than to throw a party? Celebrating Hawaii's admission to the U.S. as the 50th state was the perfect excuse to throw a luau!

They were finishing up the dance contest when I walked in. The handsome young groundskeeper was participating and helping to lead the resident dancers. One lady was awarded a special paper crown as 'Queen of the Dance' and she showed her happiness with a broad toothy smile.

Everyone had a lei of silk flowers around their neck and those dancing the hula wore grass skirts tied around their waist. Don Ho was singing from the portable CD player, streamers hung from the ceiling, transparent plastic sheets with large palm trees hung in front of the windows, and Hawaiian-themed graphics adorned the walls.

Rounding out the beautification were two unlit tiki torches, and a portable steel fire pit in the center of the room was fitted with yellow, orange, and red construction paper cut to look like flames. A big island hut, built by the residents as a craft project, was on the center of the table. It was made of brown paper lunch bags with vertical cuts along their bottoms to resemble thatch.

Tropical punch and fruit kabobs with pineapple, watermelon, and cantaloupe were served. Everyone was given a napkin with a large, brightly colored tiki face as a parting gift.

Mom sat with her eyes closed most of the time with a lei encircling her neck. Even when her eyes were open, it seemed she had no clue that there was a party going on and that the place was buzzing with activity. She sipped punch through a super-skinny straw so at least she enjoyed something.

* * *

Tuesday was Mardi Gras, and that meant there was an opportunity for the Activities Department to celebrate! A CD filled the room with the upbeat jazzy sounds of New Orleans. Purple, green, and gold paper masks were held in place with a thin string of elastic, hiding the residents faces from the nose up. They had cut outs for the eyes and jester-style hats. Necklaces made of colored beads and monochrome fish were draped around everyone's necks.

Theresa made her way around the room encouraging everyone to dance. It's a great form of exercise and I know that Mom usually participates in other dancing activities. That's no surprise since she has always loved to dance from the time she was square dancing as a teen. I remember her teaching me the "Alley Cat" and "Bunny Hop" in our living room when I was growing up.

As the AD approached us, I asked Mother Dear if she wanted to dance. The AD took my cue and took hold of Mom's hands and got her to stand. They started dancing and Theresa would lift Mom's arms and twirl under.

I watched her. Light on her feet, yet her legs lacked coordination and showed signs of their age. It was her eyes that told the whole story of her current state. Open and staring ahead. Vacant. The body was moving from something basic in her brain, but the mind wasn't, her conscious mind gone.

I left the building, got in the car, and wept.

* * *

There was a clam steam at the end of every summer. Again, each resident was allowed two guests. This shindig probably had the most attendance out of all their events.

It was a good way for us to mix with other families. It seemed we knew every resident and some of the other families, so we'd become social butterflies.

My brother and I drove up together and parked in the lot visible from the outdoor tent they'd constructed to shade the picnic tables from the sun. When we got out of the car, Mom spotted us immediately and waved. We were about 50 yards away so there was proof her eyesight was good, too. As we approached, she pointed to the car, knowing it was hers.

The weather was a bit problematic for the older folks. It was beautiful, a slight breeze blowing across the lawn, and the sky was full of large puffy cumulus clouds drifting by. Unfortunately, when the sun wasn't obstructed it was too warm. When the clouds moved in the way, it was too cool.

Mom was very sensitive to temperature so this constant changing from hot to cold made her antsy. She kept getting up, not knowing where she was going, but knowing she didn't want to sit at the table anymore because she wasn't comfortable. We tried to keep her jacket on/off but that wasn't working. Another lady, without her family, sat with us and I kept helping her do the same thing with her sweater.

Once the food began to arrive, they settled down. The staff started by serving Manhattan clam chowder with crackers. That was followed by clams in a mesh bag that had just been steamed, with a side of melted butter for dipping. The main meal consisted of boneless chicken breast, ribs, corn on the cob, and potato salad. Dessert was a slice of watermelon or cantaloupe. Mom ate some of the Chex mix that was on the table but didn't touch a bite of anything else.

A man played a guitar and sang classics like *King of the Road* as entertainment. I sang along to Mother Dear and she smiled.

We escorted Mom back to her room at 1. She was fast asleep seconds after her head hit the pillow.

THE HORSE PISTOL

Mom's physical health was quite good for a long time after being placed on the anti-seizure medication for the pain in her jaw.

Then Mother Dear had a spell while they were showering her at the assisted living center. Based on their description, it sounded similar to the other mini seizures she had at home. She would be okay within 15 minutes and I mentioned that to the nurse who called to report the incident. She confirmed that Mom was indeed feeling better already but they were going to send her to the emergency room anyway. They had to play it safe and I understood that they had to take extra precautions with the folks in their care.

I had the option of going up to the hospital (my father always called it the horse pistol), a 45 minute drive, but the nurse said she wasn't sure that they'd even admit her and she'd probably be brought back that night. Given that I'd seen this before, and that she had already come out of it before she left for the hospital, I opted to have them call me if things changed.

The emergency room doctors diagnosed her with a Urinary Tract Infection (UTI), wrote a prescription for antibiotics, and did indeed send her back that night. I called in the morning and they reported that she was back to her 'normal' self.

Over the two years she was living there, she had deteriorated to where she couldn't really talk anymore and hadn't recognized me at all over the previous two weeks. It had been a long time since she knew I was her son, or my name, but at least she'd known me as a friendly face and that I was there to see her. When dementia patients are sick, as I've mentioned, they can't really tell you so the staff is trained to watch for changes in behavior. It occurred to me that her lack of recognizing me could have been due to the UTI rather than just having a bad day or following the normal progression of the illness. I hoped she would change back to knowing me once she got on the new medication.

This incident came before she was rushed to the hospital after falling down twice within an hour. I had left her from my regular visit just two hours before and she seemed fine.

Complaining of neck pain at the emergency room, they did a CT scan, and spotted a "mass" on her thyroid. Not good. I gave approval to do an ultrasound to determine what we were dealing with. She had legal Do Not Resuscitate (DNR) paperwork and that might impact any further decisions regarding her care.

She wasn't admitted, rather sent back to the assisted living center, pending an appointment for the ultrasound.

Less than a week later I received a call at 4 a.m. that they were sending Mom to the hospital. On a bed check, they found her sitting on the edge of her mattress and she had been vomiting. When they tried to give her a shower to clean her up, she passed out several times. She was cold and clammy so they called the rescue squad.

The flu had been racing through the facility, a strain that wasn't kept at bay by that year's preventative shot. The whole place was on Tamiflu to keep them from coming down with it and they were discouraging visitors.

At the horse pistol, she didn't have a fever, tested negative for the flu, and had an elevated white cell count indicating an infection. She was complaining of stomach pain so they did another CT scan. The diagnosis was a twist in her small intestine. The recommendation was to admit her, put her on IV only, and see if it would resolve itself with bed rest. A KUB X-ray looked good so they put her on clear liquids. She hadn't thrown up since the first incident.

If it didn't resolve itself, one option was surgery. This would entail cutting her abdomen open from side to side and possibly re-sectioning the bowel. Again, we would need to wrestle with the decision to go ahead with such an invasive operation. It was questionable whether a surgeon would actually perform such a complex procedure on someone so old and frail.

We weren't sure if she would be able to return to her regular place or if they were going to move her to a nursing home. She was still weak and three days without food didn't help.

After the latest X-rays showed no bowel obstruction and her white cell count was back to normal, the medical team suspected it

IV

EPILOGUE

Everything in the will went to my brother and me as "share and share alike" — divided 50/50. We met with a lawyer to draw up the necessary paperwork for the house to be transferred to us as Tenants In Common and began taking the beneficiary distributions from her life insurance policies and investments. The government got their share.

My brother was generous and agreed to give me the sporty little Cavalier that Mother Dear had tooled around in. After 10 years, it only had 38,000 miles on the odometer. I made some much-needed repairs, put on a new set of tires, and it has been good, reliable transportation.

I am staying in the house for now, continuing my efforts to go through Mom's stuff. I go back and forth between clothes, collectibles, paperwork, trophies, and photo albums. "You can't take it with you," is certainly the truth and I find it depressing to disassemble a life that took eight decades to build.

I dropped off nearly 50 dress outfits, 20 pocketbooks, and 10 pair of shoes to Dress for Success. It is a local charity that helps needy women get on their feet with professional clothing for job interviews. The remainder of her clothes have been donated to a charity that works with the homeless, elderly, sick, and underprivileged.

Using her things to help her family and others is how Mother Dear would have liked it.

may have been some other type of flu since the assisted care facility was now rife with gastro-intestinal issues. She may have been one of the first to come down with it. An illness from which she never fully recovered.

It was a diagnosis that made sense and we agreed with — that was the good news. The bad news was that she was refusing to eat. When we were there on her last night in the horse pistol before being moved to a nursing home, my brother tried to give her some water, broth, and Jell-O with a spoon. As I watched and listened to him, it put me back to how he was with his daughters when they were babies.

Her assisted care place sent their head nurse to do an evaluation and she said they weren't equipped to handle her level of required care. She couldn't go back there, at least not then, but perhaps after getting some rehabilitation at a nursing home.

She needed to get out of the hospital and into some place where they performed that type of rehabilitation service. Her Medicare provider denied coverage on the first call. They said there wasn't any sense in covering rehab since her dementia was so advanced. Her primary physician called the insurance company's medical director and convinced them to cover her for the weekend during an evaluation period.

She went to the Rehabilitation Center and Nursing Home in Bennington, the same place her mother had spent her final days. The idea was to get her back up to speed, eating on her own and walking, and back to the assisted living facility. After the weekend we'd know if she was getting better and would be able to feed herself, if she was willing to eat but needed help, or that she wasn't going to eat at all.

Years ago my neighbor told me that her mother died from dementia two weeks after she stopped eating. Mom's doctor confirmed that was common. If she refused to eat, it was the end. We made the decision not to have anything done intravenously to keep her alive, per her wishes.

One thing that stressed us out was that we'd have to go "private pay" to get her into a nursing home due to our reliance on the LTC policy rather than Medicaid. They wanted first month plus another month security up front. That was $17,460 ($291 a day). Even though we had the policy in place, which would reimburse $250 a day, we still needed that initial chunk of change up front just to get the ball rolling with her admittance!

When we saw her next, she drifted between states of awake and sleep, showing signs of awareness when her eyes were open. She was eating and the nursing staff reported that she had been able to feed herself if the food was put in little bowls that she could manage.

She did make progress over the summer, sometimes eating on her own, sometimes forming sentences ("I have to go to the bathroom"). She kept trying to get up out of her chair and was able to stand unassisted in the shower. She could pull herself along in the wheel chair where the nurses placed her in the morning, wandering the halls and looking into all the rooms. When she got to the end of the corridor, an aide would turn her around and back she'd go to the nurses' station. She had wasted away to skin and bones but was still able to sit up and take notice of the things going on around her.

The staff called my brother on Christmas Eve to let us know she'd taken a turn for the worse. We'd received these types of calls before when she'd slid down out of her chair and "fell." After a report that she was continuing to get worse and her condition was critical, my brother went up on the day after Christmas and sat with her while I was at work.

The following morning, he came down to the house, telling me that we needed to get up to see her because she was going to die soon based on what he'd seen the previous day. The plan was to meet at his house and carpool up since the drive was long and it was best not to face the dire situation alone.

By the time I arrived at his house, my brother met me on the cracked pavement of his driveway with tears in his eyes. He'd just received the call that Mother Dear had died. We still went up to see her and I was shocked by the sight of her lying in bed. I tried to fight back the tears spilling from my eyes and rolling down over my flushed cheeks. It sounds a bit naïve but I didn't expect her to look dead. I guess I'm used to seeing dead bodies at wakes after they have been restored to their former looks.

The funeral went exactly as she wanted it. Just immediate family: me, my brother and his wife, their two daughters (Mom's granddaughters) and their fiancés, and her brother. The funeral director was the same person that had managed the services for my father. In fact, all of her burial plans matched his.

Mother Dear looked wonderful in an open shiny silver casket at the front of the room. We had her dressed all in purple because that was her favorite color. Her sweater was visible and we chose to have her buried with her glasses on since that is how she had always appeared.

We were there for an hour, from 11 a.m. to noon, during which time my uncle called my brother and me aside for a "confession." He told us that he realized he hadn't been a very good brother or uncle. I was a little uncomfortable with him relieving his conscience but I was happy that he acknowledged that his behavior had been, how shall I say, less than ideal. His years-long absence, when he was needed the most, was hurtful. He had been deeply missed and the person who really needed to hear the apology was no longer with us. Perhaps he included those thoughts in his prayers as he said his farewell.

The short service included a reading by the rector of the All Saints Episcopal church where she and her family had been congregants. Working from the back row to front, I was the first asked by the undertaker to approach her and say a final goodbye. I spent a moment looking at her, working to commit this final image of my Mother Dear to memory.

After everyone had their turn, we then braced for the cold and followed the hearse on a 20-minute journey to the cemetery. Graveside, it was 15°F and windy, making it very uncomfortable. I had prepared well, wearing thermal underwear underneath my new black suit and knee-length wool overcoat.

The funeral director did one last confirmation that Mom was being buried in the correct direction and plot location. The rector, shivering, read a few more passages taken from the Bible and his frozen breath was visible as he spoke. The ceremony complete, we took to our cars. My brother led us on our old familiar route past her childhood farm for one last time.

She is now lying along side my father, to his left, as they had stood at the altar at their wedding.

She led a good life. May she rest in peace...

www.ingramcontent.com/pod-product-compliance
Lightning Source LLC
Chambersburg PA
CBHW061506180526
45171CB00001B/53